Health, Risk and Vulnerability

The concept of risk is one of the most suggestive terms for evoking the cultural character of our times and for defining the purpose of social research. Risk attitudes and behaviours are understood to comprise the dominant experience of culture, politics and society.

Health, Risk and Vulnerability investigates the personal and political dimensions of health risk that structure everyday thought and action. In this innovative book, international contributors reflect upon the meaning and significance of risk across a broad range of social and institutional contexts, exploring current issues such as:

- the 'escalation of the medicalization of life', involving the pathologization of normality and blurring of the divide between clinical and preventive medicine
- the tendency for mental health service users to be regarded as representing a risk to others rather than being 'at risk' and vulnerable themselves
- the development of health care systems to identify risk and prevent harm
- women's reactions to 'high risk' screening results during pregnancy and how they communicate with other women about risk
- men and the use of the internet to reconstruct their social and sexual identities.

Charting new terrain in the sociology of health and risk, and focusing on the connections between them, *Health, Risk and Vulnerability* offers new perspectives on an important field of contemporary debate and provides an invaluable resource for students, teachers, researchers, and policy makers.

Alan Petersen is Professor of Sociology, School of Political and Social Inquiry, Monash University, Australia.

Iain Wilkinson is Senior Lecturer in Sociology at the School of Social Policy, Sociology and Social Research, University of Kent, UK.

Health, Risk and Vulnerability

Edited by Alan Petersen
and Iain Wilkinson

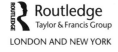
Routledge
Taylor & Francis Group

LONDON AND NEW YORK

First published 2008
by Routledge
2 Park Square, Milton Park, Abingdon, Oxon, OX14 4RN

Simultaneously published in the USA and Canada
by Routledge
270 Madison Ave, New York, NY 10016

Routledge is an imprint of the Taylor & Francis Group, an informa business

Typeset in Times by
GreenGate Publishing Services, Tonbridge, Kent

Printed and bound in Great Britain by
T J International Ltd, Padstow, Cornwall

British Library Cataloguing in Publication Data
A catalogue record for this book is available from the British Library

Library of Congress Cataloging in Publication Data
Health, risk, and vulnerability / edited by Alan Petersen and Iain Wilkinson.
p. ; cm.
Includes bibliographical references and index.
1. Health behavior. 2. Health attitudes. 3. Risk-taking (Psychology)--Social aspects.
4. Health risk assessment--Social aspects. I. Petersen, Alan R., Ph. D. II. Wilkinson,
Iain, 1969-
[DNLM: 1. Health Behavior. 2. Attitude to Health. 3. Cultural Characteristics. 4.
Health Policy. 5. Risk Management. 6. Risk-Taking. W 85 H43498 2008]
RA776.9.H45 2008
362.1--dc22
2007018244

ISBN-10: 0–415–38307–2 (hbk)
ISBN-10: 0–415–38308–0 (pbk)

ISBN-13: 978–0–415–38307–3 (hbk)
ISBN-13: 978–0–415–38308–0 (pbk)

Contents

Contributors

Andy Alaszewski is Professor of Health Studies and Director of the Centre for Health Services Research at the University of Kent. His research examines the ways in which the assessment, perception and management of risk structures the ways in which health and social care service users experience the care and support they receive. He is editor of the international journal *Health, Risk & Society*. His publications include Alaszewski, A. *et al.* (eds) (1998) *Risk, Health and Welfare: Policies, Strategies and Practice* (Open University Press) and Alaszewski, A. *et al.* (2000) *Managing Risk in Community Practice: Nursing, Risk and Decision Making* (Bailliere Tindall).

Kirstie Coxon, Research Associate, Centre for Health Services Studies (CHSS), University of Kent, is a health services researcher with a background in nursing and midwifery, and has worked on a range of projects in older people's health and social care, using a mixture of methodologies including quantitative, qualitative and case study/evaluation research. Kirstie's areas of research interest include partnership working, integrated health and social care, care of older people and primary care research. She is currently academic lead for the Kent arm of the South East Research and Development Support Unit.

Jacqueline Davies is a Research Fellow in the Health Care Research Unit at City University. She is interested in a wide range of public policy research issues. Her publications include (2002) 'The research potential of practice nurses' *Health and Social Care in the Community* 10(5): 370–81 and (2006) 'The problems of offenders with mental disorders' *Social Science and Medicine* 63: 1097–1108.

Paul Godin is a Senior Lecturer in Sociology at City University. His edited book *Risk and Nursing Practice* was published in 2006 in the Palgrave sociology and nursing practice series. He was the principal investigator on a Department of Health funded service user-led project completed in 2006, 'Engaging service users in the evaluation and development of forensic mental health care services'.

Bob Heyman is Associate Dean for Research and Professor of Health Research at St Bartholomew School of Nursing & Midwifery at City University. His research focus is qualitative approaches to health risk management. He has researched and published in relation to a wide variety of groups, including pregnant women who are offered chromosomal screening, adults with learning disabilities and forensic mental health/learning disabilities service users. His publications include Heyman, B. and Henriksen, M. (2001) *Risk, Age and Pregnancy: A Case Study of Prenatal Genetic Screening and Testing* (Palgrave) and Heyman, B. (ed.) (1998) *Risk, Health and Health Care: A Qualitative Approach* (Edward Arnold).

Pru Hobson-West is a Research Fellow based at the University of Nottingham in the Institute for Science and Society. She is currently researching issues around the use of animals in biomedical science. Her publications include (2007) 'Trusting blindly can be the biggest risk of all' *Sociology of Health & Illness* 29: 2 and (2003) 'Understanding vaccination resistance: moving beyond risk' *Health, Risk & Society* 5: 3.

Dawn S. Jones is Senior Lecturer in Sociology at Liverpool Hope University. Her research focuses on the relation between discourse, perception and reality. Her recent publications have explored the relation between expert narratives and the perception of risk. Building on her research into women's perceptions of risk in pregnancy, she is currently exploring the production of risk-knowledge amongst health care professionals. Recent and forthcoming publications include a chapter in Raisborough, J. and Scott, J. (eds) (forthcoming) *Risk, Identity & the Everyday* and in Bates, D. (2007) *Marxism, Intellectuals and Politics* (Palgrave).

Alan Petersen is Professor of Sociology at the School of Political and Social Inquiry, Monash University, Melbourne, Australia. His research encompasses the sociology of health and illness, sociology of new biomedical technologies, the sociology of risk and gender and sexuality studies. His recent publications include *The Body in Question: A Socio-Cultural Approach* (Routledge, 2007) and *Engendering Emotions* (Palgrave, 2004).

Anthony Pryce originally intended to be an art historian but is now Reader in Sociology (Sexual Health) at the Institute of Health Sciences, City University, London. His research focuses on sexualities and health in hard to reach and hidden populations. He contributes widely to the literature and recent publications include (2006) '"Let's talk about sex": Kinsey, outrage and the construction of postmodern sexualities' *Sexuality & Culture* 10(1): 63–93 and '"...planting landmines in their sex lives": governmentality, iconography of sexual disease and the "duties" of the STD clinic', in King, M. and Watson, K. (eds) (2005) *Representing Health: Discourses of Health and Illness in the Media* (Palgrave).

Lisa Reynolds is a Lecturer in Forensic Mental Health Care at City University. Her PhD is on the experience of forensic mental health care and risk management in a medium secure forensic mental health unit. She has undertaken research into forensic mental health care and risk both in the UK and South

Africa. She has forthcoming publications based on an on-line discussion forum e-learning project with mental health service users and student mental health nurses, and a women incarceration workshop.

Monica Shaw is a Senior Research Fellow at City University and was previously Dean of Social Sciences, Northumbria University. Her publications include Heyman, B. *et al.* (2004) 'Forensic mental health services as a health risk escalator: a case study of ideals and practice' *Health, Risk & Society* 6: 307–25.

John-Arne Skolbekken is an Associate Professor in Community Psychology at the Department of Psychology, the Norwegian University of Science and Technology (NTNU), in Trondheim, Norway. His research is focused on the influence of the risk concept in modern medicine and modern living. As a member of NTNU's Research Group in Bioethics, he is currently involved in research projects focusing on the impact of various forms of medical screening on lay people's health perceptions. His publications include (1995) 'The risk epidemic in medical journals' *Social Science and Medicine* 40(3): 291–305 and (1998) 'Communicating the risk reductions achieved by cholesterol reducing drugs' *BMJ* 316: 1956–8.

Joost Van Loon is Professor of Media Analysis at the Institute of Cultural Analysis, Nottingham Trent University. His current research focuses on media technologies, risk, affect and sense-perceptions, among other things. He is co-editor of the journal *Space and Culture*. His recent publications include *Risk and Technological Culture: Towards a Sociology of Virulence* (Routledge, 2002). He is currently finishing a monograph entitled *Media Technologies: An Introduction to Media Analysis* (Open University Press).

Joanne Warner is a Senior Lecturer in Social Work in the School of Social Policy, Sociology and Social Research, University of Kent. Her research interests include socio-cultural approaches to risk, mental health and social work and the significance of 'race' and ethnicity, gender and place in this context. She has also explored the impact of cultures of inquiry and blame on professional practice. Recent publications include Warner, J. and Gabe, J. 'Risk, mental disorder and social work practice: a gendered landscape' *British Journal of Social Work* Advance Access, 17 October 2006 and Warner, J. (2006) 'Inquiry reports as active texts and their function in relation to professional practice in mental health' *Health, Risk & Society* 8(3): 223–37.

Iain Wilkinson is a Senior Lecturer in Sociology in the School of Social Policy, Sociology and Social Research, University of Kent. His research explores socio-cultural approaches to risk and contemporary forms of 'social suffering'. His work engages with social theory, the sociology of risk, the sociology of health and the history of sociology. His publications include *Anxiety in a Risk Society* (Routledge, 2001) and *Suffering: A Sociological Introduction* (Polity Press, 2005).

Abbreviations

AA	Alcoholics Anonymous
AAA	Action Against Autism
AiA	Allergy induced Autism
ASW	approved social worker
BMJ	*British Medical Journal*
CDA	critical discourse analysis
CHD	coronary heart disease
CMC	computer-mediated communication
GM	genetically modified
GUM	Genito-Urinary Medicine
HRA	Health Risk Appraisal
JABS	Justice Awareness and Basic Support
JFAVDC	Justice for All Vaccine Damaged Children
MMR	measles, mumps and rubella
MSU	medium secure unit
PICU	Psychiatric Intensive Care Unit
PMS	premenstrual syndrome
RCT	randomized controlled trial
SAHM	stay-at-home mum
SARF	Social Amplification of Risk Framework
STI	sexually transmitted infection
TPS	Teenage Pregnancy Strategy
VAN	Vaccine Awareness Network

Chapter 1

Health, risk and vulnerability

An introduction

Alan Petersen and Iain Wilkinson

The concept of risk is now well established as part of the language of social science. It is widely accepted that the experience of everyday life is significantly influenced by the ways in which individuals think and act about and institutions respond to 'risk'. Encounters with risk are perceived to take place within every aspect of our public and private lives. Indeed, it has become almost a matter of sociological common sense to identify risk as both an organising principle of society and a major coordinate of personal identity. Risk now features as one of the most suggestive terms for evoking the cultural character of our times and for defining the purpose of social research.

Yet there is no agreement among the social science community as to why risk has come to occupy such a central position within the terms of academic and public debate. Broadly speaking, there are at least four contrasting ways in which analysts venture to explain this interest. Firstly, following Ulrich Beck, an emphasis has been placed upon the extent to which the public salience of risk signals that people are increasingly aware that technological hazards and industrial pollutants are drawing us to the brink of ecological catastrophe (Beck 1992). Accordingly, our shared interest in risk is framed as an expression of the fact that we know ourselves to be living in an environment made dangerous through the hazards courted by modern science and technology. A second explanation is developed with reference to Mary Douglas' cultural theory, where it is argued that the popularisation of risk is more closely related to a pronounced experience of individualisation in modern societies that erodes traditional ties of moral solidarity and community (Douglas 1985, 1992). On this account, it is not so much the case that we know for sure that the reality of danger is increasing; but rather, via an erosion of trust in public institutions we are made to be more anxiously disposed to express our concerns in terms of 'risk'. Thirdly, an accent has been placed upon the 'stigmatisation' that results from the way in which modern science tends to be portrayed in mass media (Flynn *et al.* 2001). This is perceived to be further exacerbated by a common psychological tendency to exaggerate the threat of dangers we associate with institutions and technologies that are beyond our immediate sphere of influence and control (Slovic 2000). Fourthly, basing their work on a critical analysis of the language of current government legislation and social policy, some claim that, if we are more prone to address our motives, attitudes and experiences in terms of risk, then this is the result of a governmental strategy that is designed to promote 'individual responsibility' as the organising ethos of welfare and work (O'Malley 2004; Rose 1999).

A considerable conflict of interpretations surrounds the social significance and political meaning of risk in our times. In this chapter we take the view that any reference to risk needs to be carefully qualified so as to make clear the analytical frame in which it is set. From the outset of our discussion, we emphasise that, in the context of social science and health studies, the language of risk comes ready laden with theoretical premises, ethical commitments and political interests. We are critical of any attempt to present 'risk' as simply another word for a 'problem' or form of 'precautionary deliberation' or 'probabilistic thinking', for we recognise this concept to be embedded in cultural worldviews that present us with *ideologically* stylised accounts of our society, individuality and the moral ties that bind us.

Our particular interest lies in the associations and conjunctions between health, risk and vulnerability. We follow a number of writers in arguing that, whilst it is widely acknowledged that the meaning of 'health' has been revolutionised over the last fifty years so that the 'healthy person' is now readily identified as engaged in the pursuit of ideal conditions of physical and mental well-being, then this was always bound to make 'health' a matter of negotiation with 'risk'. We understand the cultural practices, social techniques and institutional arrangements that are now committed to the pursuit of health to be heavily implicated in the current popularisation of the language of risk. Indeed, we go so far as to suggest that, more often than not, where the politics of risk becomes a public concern, then at the same time this is bound to the politics of health; and where we aim to expose the ideological interests at work within the language of risk, we are also concerned to bring critical attention to the ideological construction of our notions of health, health practice and health promotion.

The politics of health risk gives rise to debate over the definition, bounds and meaning of human vulnerability, and in recent years this matter has been brought to the fore across a number of fields of interest. Most notably it features in development and disaster studies as a means to draw critical debate towards the plight of the most materially and institutionally disadvantaged groups in developing societies (Blaickie *et al.* 1994). In these domains, it is often the case that reference to people's 'vulnerability' takes place as writers work to criticise technocratic approaches to risk and disaster management that overlook the involvement of state policy and capital interests in the on-set of disaster. Accordingly, by highlighting the ways in which populations are made 'vulnerable' to experience harms, either challenges are brought to the ways in which the causes of disasters are officially identified (i.e. as discrete events that 'strike' from 'outside' the normal workings of the status quo) or, rather, increased levels of vulnerability are identified as the unintended consequence of managerial policy. At the same time, the concept of vulnerability features as part of a new managerial discourse that aims to target sectors of population for policy intervention (Alwang *et al.* 2001; Delor and Hubert 2000). Accordingly, while on the one hand reference to human vulnerability is used as a means to caution against the ways in which technical regimes of risk management are blind to the human consequences of regulatory practice, on the other hand it is being adopted as part of a technical language that is designed to specify problems for increased measures of expert intervention and technological control. One way or another, it appears that expert approaches to risk assessment and practices of risk management are having the unanticipated effect of making the appeal to human vulnerability a major component of debates over the legitimacy of government and governmental technologies of risk.

We contend that it is increasingly the case that the discourse on human vulnerability features heavily in critical debates over the bounds of 'health risk' in so-called 'advanced' industrial societies. In this regard, the sociology of health risk appears to be mirroring developments in disaster and development studies. However, one noticeable difference concerns the extent to which the debates on vulnerability in countries such as Britain and the United States are not simply focused on questions of survival and basic needs, but rather encompass concerns such as the felt quality of patient–practitioner interactions and emotional well-being of individuals. In the context of Western medicine, the turn to debates on vulnerability reflects an ever-broadening conception of health as well as the tendency to subsume health under the category of risk.

Constructing 'health' in terms of 'risk'

In modern times, the conceptualisation of health has been transformed to a point where commentators are prone to take this as an indication of a paradigm shift in the common experience of embodiment, self and society. From 1947 onwards, definitions of health advanced and elaborated by the World Health Organization are held up as a collective representation of a new approach to thinking about human well-being that, rather than locate this as simply a matter of bodily function, emphasises the extent to which our capacity to feel healthy takes place as a mode of interaction between body, culture and society. Whilst a Cartesian approach towards understanding the body persists within many sectors of medical research and practice, increasingly this is supplemented and challenged by a more 'holistic' account of health that places emphasis upon the extent to which our felt quality of life is determined by social environment and cultural outlook (Larson 1999).

In part, this development can be attributed to improvements in material conditions, coupled with advances in medical science, which have radically transformed patterns of morbidity and mortality among Western populations. Here the majority of people no longer die from tuberculosis, diarrhoea and pneumonia, but rather from heart disease, cancer and stroke. Towards the end of the nineteenth century and during the first half of the twentieth century, dramatic improvements in bodily health and quality of life were achieved through sanitation, nutrition, vaccination campaigns and antibiotic treatments. Throughout this time, the principal causes of disease could be identified among a discrete range of environmental and biological factors, for which it was possible to specify effective solutions and treatments. This was the era of 'magic-bullet' medicine, which according to Allan Brandt encouraged the popular understanding of health as the absence of a clearly identifiable disease (Brandt 1997). However, in a context where the most life-threatening disease is not so much 'caught', but 'acquired', a new epidemiology has emerged that emphasises a host of environmental, social and behavioural factors that hitherto were not recognised by medical science as a health concern.

The association of 'health' with 'risk' is encouraged by the epidemiological understanding that many of the most life-threatening diseases are caused through a combination of multiple lifestyle factors. David Armstrong contends that the language of risk enters into the everyday lexicon of medical practice at the point where the imperatives of health care move beyond the treatment of bodily symptoms to work at understanding and controlling social environments implicated within the aetiology of modern 'diseases of affluence' (Armstrong 1995: 400). Health care as 'risk management' is an integral feature of 'surveillance medicine'; it amounts to a further intensification and extension of processes of rationalisation around the conduct of the individual and social body. It emerges when medical researchers turn to biostatistics and randomised controlled trials as the means to identify segments of population most 'at risk' of developing symptoms of disease. Indeed, John-Arne Skolbekken maintains that it was particularly in the aftermath of the application of computing technologies to the gathering and analysis of probability statistics relating to health and illness that the language risk reached 'epidemic' proportions in medical journals (Skolbekken 1995: 298).

This development was further consolidated by the rise of 'health promotion' as a distinct field of clinical practice (Lupton 1995; Petersen and Lupton 1996). However, it is important to note that here the vested interests in matters of risk move beyond technical problems of calculation; for the language of risk is also strategically employed in attempts to promote positive health behaviours. Alongside the actuarial understanding of risk that features within practices of 'Health Risk Appraisal' (HRA) as promoted by the Society for Prospective Medicine, and the World Health Organization's 'Risk Approach' framework, there is also a move to advance forms of moral judgement on the health-related aspects of people's lifestyles. Following Mary Douglas, many writers note that, in popular usage, the word 'risk' is used as a synonym for danger; and further, that a danger identified as 'risk' is redolent with moral meaning. 'Risk' is used both to highlight a potential harm and to identify the sources of danger. The labelling of attitudes and behaviours as 'risk' implies a negative judgement upon how these are formed and take place. Accordingly, a number of writers work to make clear the ways the language of risk is now being used to apportion moral responsibility and blame (Douglas 1992; Joffe 1999). Where attitudes and behaviours are labelled as risk and where institutions and individuals complain that they are 'at risk', then this is intended as a form of moral censure. Here an emphasis is placed upon risk as wholly 'undesirable' and as always involving a call for some manner of intervention to take place so as to correct, reform and morally rectify those outlooks and actions implicated within the possibility of harm.

Some examples of the dual character of risk can be found in studies conducted by Bob Heyman and Mette Henriksen into the communication of information relating to possible hazards associated with prenatal genetic testing for older women (Henriksen and Heyman 1998; Heyman and Henriksen 1998). Here they detail the various ways in which risks are presented to women so as to both communicate the probabilities related to the genetic screening for Down's syndrome and the bounds of moral responsibility in discussions between health practitioners and women over the circumstances where the latter might choose to terminate a pregnancy. Whilst documenting the potential for medical experts to communicate probabilities so as to guide women towards the decisions that suit their professional and institutional interests, Henriksen and Heyman also note that, in many instances, pregnant women appeared to be influenced more by the moral meaning of risk, than by matters of statistical quantification. For the women concerned, it was not so much due to the insights gained through probabilistic reasoning, but more through a process of negotiation with the social stigma of being identified as courting possible risks, that they decided whether or not to subject themselves to serum screening or an amniocentesis.

Indeed, in many studies of the social representation of health risks, a greater emphasis is placed on the extent to which people are more likely to respond to risk with a display of anxiety, rather than take this as a cue to exercise more control over their lives. For example, Nina Hallowell and colleagues argue that, whilst the expert categorisation of health-related behaviours in terms of risk takes place with the aim of extending domains of technical control over the body so as to extend life and minimise harm, in many instances this serves to have a negative impact upon people's emotional well-being (Hallowell 1999; Hallowell *et al.* 2004). In their studies of women attending genetic counselling and testing for hereditary breast cancer, they found that respondents suffered considerable amounts of distress when presented with information on their chances of developing the disease. Whilst patients set out with the original intention of better managing their future health, the increased knowledge of risk acquired through their encounters with medical practitioners became a source of considerable anxiety so that, rather than developing an enhanced sense of control over their lives, they became increasing fatalistic about their life chances.

Accordingly, in the conjunction of health with risk we are presented with the paradox that, whilst this might be readily associated with technological developments and social practices that are designed to increase powers of control over the human body and hazards of life, at the level of everyday experience it may serve more to heighten people's sense of vulnerability before the contingencies of life. Where, on the one hand, the professional discourse of risk can be framed as a set of ritualised practices for managing collective anxieties relating to ever more elaborated domains of modern medicine and health care, on the other hand they can be viewed as having the unintended consequence of further intensifying shared feelings of insecurity before future uncertainties (Crawford 2004; Wilkinson 2001). By working to control for the future, the unwitting result is that the future is made to appear more menacing.

Arguably, this paradox is further complicated by the ways in which the language of risk is mobilised as a major component of campaigns for health promotion. Where efforts are made to worry people into giving up smoking, lowering their consumption of alcohol, eating a more balanced diet or practising safe sex, then the popular association of risk with danger is readily courted and emphasised. While expert understandings of risk are framed in terms of probabilistic reason, calculation and control, risk is often dramatised as danger for the purpose of promoting good health behaviours. The actuarial account of risk in terms of a technical assessment of probabilities is always liable to be coloured by a more emotive meaning of risk as vulnerability and danger. Further, we find health professionals using the language in both ways according to the guiding interests of their work (Heyman 1998). On these grounds, the language of risk is increasingly made the focus of ideological debate and political controversy.

The ideology and politics of risk

Risk is central to the workings of politics and power in many contemporary societies and provides a major focus for ideological debate in various fields apart from health care and public health, including crime, delinquency, unemployment and the homeless. The so-called 'new' public health is indicative of this emphasis, with its concern about risks in physical and social environments and personal behaviours and about the means to their prevention (Petersen and Lupton 1996). As the contributors to this book emphasise, risk always presupposes some preventive intervention. The epidemiology of 'risk' has led to preventive strategies on a range of fronts, from the global level (e.g. World Health Organization immunisation programmes) to the individual level (e.g. the self-policing of sexual conduct). Health promotion has developed a battery of strategies for identifying and countering 'unhealthy' or 'risky' lifestyles (Hansen and Easthope 2007: 16–25; Petersen and Lupton 1996: 15).

In medicine, genetic and other diagnostic tests allow diagnosis of individuals 'at risk' and the creation of new categories of the 'pre-symptomatic ill'. Diagnostic technologies mean that 'Anything and everything is "sick" or can actually or potentially make one "sick" – quite independently of how a person actually feels' (Beck 1992: 205) (see chapter by Skolbekken). The self-management of risk has become an imperative of citizenship, with individuals expected to become 'knowledgeable' about the sources, nature and consequences of risk and, where possible, take appropriate preventive action. This entails the close monitoring and regulation of one's thoughts and actions and recognising oneself as 'vulnerable'. 'Risk' generates fear in relation to particular practices (e.g. the use of salt in cooking, sedentary lifestyles) and populations (e.g. the diseased and mentally ill – see chapters by Warner and Davies *et al.*). Many practices and inter-actions that were once seen as bringing pleasure have become the source of worry. The language of risk implies that a clear delineation can be made between the sources or the perpetrators of danger and sites of vulnerability or the victims. All manner of interventions into bodies and lives and all kinds of exclusions and con-trols have been legitimised on the basis that a certain behaviour, group or population presents a 'risk to society'.

Robert Castel (1991) has observed the significance of a shift 'from dangerous-ness to risk' for social regulation in contemporary societies. As he argues, the calculation of risks permits interventions to be legitimated not on the basis of actual existing dangers but rather on the basis of expert assessment that an unde-sirable event may occur and that this can be prevented through intervention (Castel 1991: 288). There is less dependence on therapeutic or corrective interventions than in the past and more emphasis on the probabilistic calculation of risk and the creation of risk profiles. Risk profiling and risk factor analyses enable the simu-lated surveillance of entire populations oriented to the fulfilment of the ideal of 'control before the event' (Bogard 1996). This includes measures to prevent dis-ease, for example the outbreak of pandemic flu (e.g. Avian flu virus), dependence on welfare (e.g. screening of immigrants and refugees) and self-harm or harm to others (e.g. screening of certain presumed mentally unstable or violent groups).

The media, including the print news media, the broadcast media, Internet, magazines, and so on, occupy a key position at the interface between expert and lay publics and are likely to exert a significant influence on responses to issues such as the above (Anderson *et al.* 2005). While it is widely recognised that the media shape or very likely do shape opinions and influence policies there is less consensus about the mechanisms of media production and the nature and extent of media influence on particular policies and viewpoints. Naïve perspectives on the workings of the media persist, despite a growing social science literature in this field. Perspectives are dominated by the Social Amplification of Risk Framework (SARF) which suggests that the media are prone to dramatisation, distortion, misrepresentation and error (Pidgeon *et al.* 2003), and work to mag-nify existing anxieties about certain phenomena. In our view, this is a simplistic 'media effects' perspective on risk mediation that greatly underestimates the vari-ety and complexity of the possible forms of interaction that take place between media, society, culture and politics (Wilkinson 1999).

With a perceived decline of trust in public confidence in authorities and in reg-ulatory systems, including those established to govern technological and other risks, this lacuna in understanding about the role of news media is surprising. Recent public debate and reactions to genetically modified crops, cloning and embryonic stem cell research indicate that news media may play a decisive influ-ence in establishing the framework for debate and policy, particularly during the early phase of the public visibility of issues, and thereby help engender the condi-tions for trust or mistrust. In the field of environmental risk, this has been shown to be the case with issues such as oil spills, industrial pollution, and climate change (see e.g. Allan *et al.* 2000). News media are full of stories of health risks and contending claims about their nature, sources, immediate impacts and longer term implications. However, although many studies have explored media portrayals of health risk, relatively little is known about the extent to which these may shape views and actions at the individual and collective level and how, in turn, widely shared visions and concerns may be reflected in the coverage of issues. News media portrayals of biotechnology, for instance, are rich with metaphors of risk which reflect the fears and fantasies that are attached to this field (Petersen 2005). Analyses of news media's framing of specific issues may provide rich insight into the cultural anxieties of our age and the vulnerabilities of particular groups.

At the time of writing, the UK Joint Committee on Human Rights, comprising MPs and peers, has voiced concerns about the mental bill on the grounds that 'vulnerable groups may end up being detained despite posing no risk to themselves or others' (Campbell 2007: 15). A news report cited the Committee's Chairman: 'The Bill proposes to change the grounds for a person's detention from "a true mental disorder" to "any disorder or disability of the mind". We are concerned that this...could result in discrimination on grounds of sexual orientation and sexual identity.' In this case, as in others, a redefinition of a category of problematic condition or behaviour can operate to widen surveillance and the potential for the regulation of certain populations. Those deemed to be 'a risk' or 'at risk' are vulnerable to having their freedoms curtailed, be subject to close monitoring, ostracism (e.g. deportation) or in some cases physical restraint (e.g. placed in quarantine). Efforts to regulate the sources of risk, the perpetrators of risk and the vulnerable, however, often engender resistance, may have unintended effects and be prone to failure or 'near misses' (see chapter by Alaszewski and Coxon).

The onset of the HIV/AIDS epidemic in the early 1980s highlighted some of the diverse implications of the politics of risk and vulnerability, with initial government and medical responses strongly focused on the supposed sources of infection and 'risky' identities and practices in the gay community and the 'policing of desire' (Watney 1997). This definition of 'the problem' led to the surveillance and the blaming of gay communities and to the further pathologisation of same-sex relations. It led policy makers to overlook the necessity to target safe-sex information at men who have sex with other men but do not self-identify as 'gay' (Jagose 1996: 19–20). Over the last few decades, the identification of the sources of risk and the tracking of populations at risk enabled by new tools of epidemiology have justified the implementation of a vast array of new measures for ensuring 'the public good', such as immunisation (e.g. MMR), fluoridation of water supplies, the regulation of food standards, and the use of quarantine for 'dangerous' groups. In each case, there has been some unintended effect, some degree of resistance and, sometimes, a failure of policy.

While we would not wish to deny the personal and collective benefits that have in the past or may in the future derive from the pursuit of certain risk management strategies, one should not lose sight of the implications of these measures including the implied personal imperatives and the resulting inequalities and exclusions.

The redefinition of 'health' in terms of 'risk' corresponds with a substantially changed relationship between citizens and expertise, with the individual called upon to take an active ongoing role in managing their relationship to risk (Rose 1990, 1999). Within the traditional biomedical conception of health, the patient is generally assumed to be passive (i.e. adopts the sick role): they hand control to the expert-practitioner who helps them get 'better' through a prescribed (and usually time-limited) course of treatment. With the growing prominence of 'risk' in health care and a general emphasis on care of the self, 'health' becomes an unfinished project, in need of constant vigilance and hard work. The 'patient' is conceived as an autonomous (i.e. unconstrained) rational seeker and 'informed consumer' of health care advice. 'Empowerment' is seen to derive from exercising 'freedom of choice' – a catchphrase that permeates policies and programmes of the NHS and other health care systems. According to a British Department of Health policy statement, 'Giving patients more choice about how, when and where they receive treatment is one cornerstone of the Government's health strategy. Another is giving members of the public a bigger hand in shaping local care systems' (http://www.dh.gov.uk/PolicyAndGuidance/PatientChoice/fs/en) (accessed 30 January 2006).

This articulation of 'choice' suggests full knowledge of options and unlimited alternatives, and denies the constraints posed by time, unequal access to resources and differences in individuals' backgrounds, propensities and abilities. Being an 'informed consumer' presupposes a range of skills and dispositions and often entails hard work. The limits of this consumer-oriented approach to health care, particularly for especially vulnerable groups such as those with mental and physical disabilities, has become evident with the recent emphasis on health care rationing, privatisation of services, competitive tendering, and so on (Henderson and Petersen 2002). A number of the chapters in this volume document examples of the enactment of this active citizenship and some of the associated and largely unacknowledged implications, in individuals' use of the Internet for networking (see chapters by Jones and Pryce) and patient groups' mobilisation against public health measures (see chapter by Hobson-West). In the marketplace, the individual is likely to be confronted with an overwhelming array of options, imperfect knowledge and conflicting advice. The language of 'choice' carries the implication that responsibility for health decisions – including for decisions 'poorly' made – lies squarely with the individual. Responsibility implies accountability and potentially blame and, in a context in which diverse information is increasingly available (though not uniformly accessible) and treatments routine, individuals are liable to being blamed and stigmatised for making the 'wrong choice'; for example, not availing themselves of particular advice or a drug or a test.

The complexities of 'consumer choice' have become especially evident with the burgeoning number of new biomedical technologies, such as prenatal genetic screening, and new drugs and devices. Genetic and other diagnostic technologies (e.g. MRI, colonoscopies) are promoted on the basis that by allowing diagnosis of risk they will enhance patient choice: individuals who are 'at risk' will be able to change their lifestyles and plan their lives with greater certainty, take the appropriate drug or treatment, or terminate a pregnancy where the risk of passing on a genetic condition to offspring is judged to be high. However, genetic and other diagnostic information can sometimes be complex and difficult to interpret, experts may disagree about the significance of test results, and in some cases the results of diagnostic tests can be more confusing than helpful (Feldman 1996). It is in examining actual examples of health care practice such as these and those in this book that the fallacy of absolute control through risk management and the limitations and implications of 'free choice' become obvious. Employing a range of perspectives and methods, the chapters explore how the discourses of risk may shape interactions in different contexts and highlight some of the uncertainties that arise from strategies of risk management. In bringing together this collection, our intention is to draw attention to the often-unacknowledged sociocultural and political significance of 'risk' in the field of health and health care. In particular, we aim to advance understanding of the conjunction of 'health', 'risk' and 'vulnerability' and of the significance of how these categories are configured for how we live our lives.

Outline of the chapters

In Chapter 2, John-Arne Skolbekken opens the discussion by documenting what he describes as 'an escalation of the medicalization of life', involving the pathologisation of normality and blurring of the divide between clinical and preventive medicine. The process of medicalisation whereby non-medical problems are transformed into medical problems has been noted by earlier writers such as Peter Conrad (Conrad and Schneider 1992). However, as Skolbekken argues, the rationality of risk takes this process further by allowing the identification and targeting of new categories of people without symptoms. Risk discourse entails new forms of surveillance and generates a heightened sense of vulnerability within the population. It is in this context that new developments such as the Polypill – a drug aimed at reducing the risk factors for cardiovascular disease – are seen to have useful application. In the chapter, Skolbekken discusses the impact and some implications of escalating medicalisation, including resistance from patients and from practitioners.

In Chapter 3, Joanne Warner examines a shift in the discourse of risk as it pertains to mental illness; namely, the tendency for mental health service users to be regarded as representing 'a risk' to others rather than being 'at risk' and vulnerable. This representation permeates both policy and media coverage of particular cases such as that involving Christopher Clunis. As Warner explains, a corollary of this shift is that 'the community' is posited as vulnerable to random attacks by strangers with mental illness. In the chapter, Warner discusses the findings of a study involving social workers from an inner-city social services department in England in the mid to late 1990s. The social workers saw themselves as taking a mediating role between service users and a fearful community; as being held responsible for managing emergent risks and for 'protecting society'. Further, risk was also closely associated with groups with specific characteristics, of a certain age, gender, 'race' and ethnicity, with black men diagnosed with schizophrenia providing a particular threat. Long-standing stereotypes about the dangers posed by young black men seemed to persist. However, it was found that professionals working in multidisciplinary teams may have different assessments of the same information about risk reflecting differences of ideology and conceptions of vulnerability. Warner concludes her chapter by arguing for the need for alternative visions of mental health and community care that challenge the current focus of policies and practices, including new alliances between and within service user movements and groups of practitioners.

In Chapter 4, Joost Van Loon focuses on another field of contemporary anxiety, namely teenage pregnancy. Drawing on the Foucaultian concept of governmentality, Van Loon critically examines the discourse of teenage sexual risk behaviour as it has been deployed by the British government in its 'Teenage Pregnancy Strategy' (TPS). As he explains, governmentality entails modes of subjugation, whereby subjects – in this case, young people – are rendered 'vulnerable' and hence in need of scrutiny and surveillance. This serves to undermine young people's integrity as subjects. An interesting paradox in the governance of teenage sexual pregnancy is that policies continue to be pursued without modification despite their evident failure: teenage pregnancies have been only minimally reduced and other indicators of sexual risk behaviour, such as sexually transmitted infections, are rising. In the chapter, Van Loon examines a number of assumptions underlying the TPS, provides evidence of its failure, and offers an explanation of why policies have been neither reconsidered nor modified despite this failure.

In Chapter 5, Andy Alaszewski and Kirstie Coxon examine the development of systems to identify risk and prevent harm in health care in the UK. As the authors indicate, the development of the regulatory state has been influenced by an enquiry culture in which accidents are classified as 'man-made' disasters; as failures to foresee and prevent risks. A series of highly publicised disasters beginning in the late 1960s and early 1970s in low-tech sectors of health and social services and then in the 1980s and 1990s in the high-tech environments of district general hospitals (including, crucially, the Bristol Royal Infirmary case) laid the foundation for the development of a new risk management regime within the health care sector. Increasingly, efforts have been made to restore trust in the regulatory systems governing medicine and other expertise. It is in this context that clinical governance, involving guidelines for the formal assessment and management of risk, and new systems for reporting adverse clinical events and 'near misses', emerged. This has necessitated a change in culture and a collaborative approach in the development of working practices. However, as the authors discovered, in their interviews with managers and professionals in one NHS organisation, a joint NHS and social care trust providing services for vulnerable adults (i.e. adults with mental illness or learning disability and older people with dementia), a lack of consensus in the framing of issues and the purpose of reporting systems for 'near misses', and professional self-interest, stymied efforts to develop an effective reporting system.

In Chapter 6, Jacqueline Davies, Paul Godin, Bob Heyman, Lisa Reynolds and Monica Shaw explore risk management in forensic mental health services employing Orne's concept of ecological validity. Ecological validity refers to the common observation that people's behaviour in the artificial conditions of the laboratory experiment cannot be generalised to everyday life and that individuals will seek to understand the purpose of the experiment and then either comply with or subvert it. The chapter draws up data from a qualitative study of risk assessment in a medium secure unit (MSU) to illustrate how ecological validity is managed by forensic services when assessing whether a service user can be assessed as being of lower risk. The study takes place against a background of a shift in mental health care policy, with an increasing emphasis on risk profiling and risk management rather than incarceration in asylums. In the chapter, the authors describe how interactions are negotiated in the MSU, in particular how service users seek to 'second guess' the intentions of staff and how both staff and service users may seek to control their respective presentations of self in order to achieve control over interactions. As the authors indicate, the impact of this new risk management regime on both service users and service providers in the field of mental health is profound, and presents lessons for risk management in other areas.

The last three chapters focus explicitly on citizens' various responses to perceptions of risk and risk information, especially via the use of the Internet, and organised opposition to policies based on risk information. In Chapter 7, Dawn Jones examines women's reactions to 'high risk' screening results during pregnancy and how they communicate with other women about risk. Her focus is the interface between 'objective' scientifically defined and validated definitions of risk and 'lay' or 'subjective' knowledge about risk and, in particular, how the latter may unsettle the former. Drawing on data from a study involving covert participation observation in an Internet antenatal 'club' oriented to women whose babies were all due in the same month (the reasons for employing this method are explained), Jones discusses women's conversations surrounding one poster's antenatal screening results. The screening test provides a 'risk calculation' in relation to carrying a foetus with Down's syndrome. The study provides interesting insights into how the women make sense of risk information and seek to offer support and reassurance to other women who are deemed to be 'at risk'. The chapter discusses the 'coping strategies' adopted by women and also the ways in which vulnerable individuals negotiate and seek to challenge objective classifications of risk. However, as Jones argues, the extent to which such challenge offers a threat to the biomedical establishment and its language of risk can be questioned. The chapter concludes with some reflections on the significance of risk information, such as that derived from antenatal screening tests, within *reflexive modernisation*.

In Chapter 8, Anthony Pryce investigates men's use of Internet chatrooms for erotic activities. It describes their interactions and how they use the Internet to reconstruct their social and sexual identities. As Pryce explains, the Internet provides new opportunities for exploring one's own sexual identities through offering an apparently 'risk-free' rehearsal space for enacting one's desires; however, there are risks involved in online encounters of this kind. It is disruptive of the heteronormative social order and it makes one vulnerable to stigmatising disclosure. Cybersex is pathologised and constructed as an addiction that can be treated like other addictions. Drawing on data from 'real-time' electronic interviews and using the work of Michel Foucault and various cyber researchers, Pryce presents a nuanced account of men's experiences of online sex. He charts the different career trajectories of different online identities (bi-curious, bisexual and gay) and the different constructions of risk and discretion management that they demand. As Pryce concludes, learning how to tell a sexual story and to test and rehearse a 'borrowed' identity involves learning the intricate expectations of both Internet communities and 'offline' society, including strategies for disguise and disclosure. Online sex involves novel forms of sociability and socialisation, an understanding of which is valuable for sociologists of health, particularly in understanding actors' 'offline' behaviours.

Finally, in Chapter 9 Pru Hobson-West explores organised resistance to a health risk strategy, namely vaccination. While a number of chapters, particularly Chapters 6, 7 and 8, examine individuals' negotiations and resistances in 'risky' situations or responses to risk information or risk profiling, this chapter focuses on *collective* opposition to a policy of risk management or prevention. As Hobson-West points out, vaccination has been posited as the bedrock of preventive medicine in that it is seen as largely responsible for declines in infectious diseases, such as polio, measles, mumps and rubella. The chapter draws on data from an interview-based study of parental groups who are opposed to vaccination in the UK, such as those opposed to MMR (measles, mumps and rubella) vaccination. Hobson-West offers some interesting reflections upon her role in the research process, given that the groups were keen to convince the researcher of the logic of their argument and to achieve publicity for their activities. Rather than adopting a realist approach to risk – which presumes that risks can be objectively measured and communicated (though perhaps not 'rationally' understood by publics) – Hobson-West conceives risks as socially constructed. This places emphasis on the sociocultural context of risk assessment and the constructed nature of 'risk' itself. In her study, she explored the discourses of groups that are critical of vaccination (Vaccine Critical groups). The chapter discusses the various ways in which risk is constructed by these groups and also how the groups challenge the dominant narratives of success. Underlying this reframing of risk, Hobson-West concludes, is a questioning of faith in science and professional expertise. She concludes, appropriately, by drawing some implications for the relationship between risk and trust in contemporary society and for the legitimacy of risk management policies such as vaccination.

References

Allan, S., Adam, B. and Carter, C. (eds) (2000) *Environmental Risks and the Media*. London and New York: Routledge.

Alwang, J., Siegel, P.B. and Jorgensen, S.L. (2001) 'Vulnerability: A view from different disciplines', *Social Protection Discussion Paper No.0015*. Washington: The World Bank.

Anderson, A., David, M., Petersen, A. and Allan, S. (2005) 'Communication or spin? Source-media relations in science journalism', in S. Allan (ed.) *Critical Issues in Journalism*. Buckingham: Open University Press.

Armstrong, D. (1995) 'The rise of surveillance medicine', *Sociology of Health & Illness* 17(3): 393–404.

Beck, U. (1992) *Risk Society: Towards a New Modernity*. London: Sage.

Blaickie, P., Cannon, T., Davis, I. and Wisner, B. (1994) *At Risk: Natural Hazards, People's Vulnerability and Disasters*. London: Routledge.

Bogard, W. (1996) *The Simulation of Surveillance: Hypercontrol in Telematic Societies*. Cambridge: Cambridge University Press.

Brandt, A.M. (1997) 'Behaviour, disease and health in the twentieth-century United States', in A.M. Brandt and P. Rozin (eds) *Morality and Health*. New York: Routledge.

Campbell, D. (2007) 'MPs voice health bill concerns', *The Observer*, February 4, p. 15.

Castel, R. (1991) 'From dangerousness to risk', in G. Burchell, C. Gordon and P. Miller (eds) *The Foucault Effect: Studies in Governmentality*. Hemel Hempstead: Harvester Wheatsheaf.

Conrad, P. and Schneider, J.W. (1992) *Deviance and Medicalization: From Badness to Sickness*, expanded edn. Philadelphia, PA: Temple University Press.

Crawford, R. (2004) 'Risk ritual and the management of control anxiety in medical culture', *Health* 8(4): 505–23.

Delor, F. and Hubert, M. (2000) 'Revisiting the concept of vulnerability', *Social Science and Medicine* 50: 1557–70.

Douglas, M. (1985) *Risk Acceptability According to the Social Sciences*. New York: Russell Sage Foundation.

Douglas, M. (1992) *Risk and Blame: Essays in Cultural Theory*. London: Routledge.

Feldman, M.K. (1996) 'Genetic screening: Not just another blood test', *Minnesota Medicine* 79: 14–17.

Flynn, J., Slovic, P. and Kunreuther, H. (eds) (2001) *Risk, Media and Stigma: Understanding Public Challenges to Modern Science and Technology*. London: Earthscan.

Hallowell, N. (1999) 'Doing the right thing: Genetic risk and responsibility', *Sociology of Health & Illness* 21(5): 597–621.

Hallowell, N., Foster, C., Eeles, R., Arden-Jones, A. and Watson, M. (2004) 'Accommodating risk: Responses to BRCA1/2 genetic testing of women who have had cancer', *Social Science and Medicine* 59: 553–65.

Hansen, E. and Easthope, G. (2007) *Lifestyle in Medicine*. London and New York: Routledge.

Henderson, S. and Petersen, A. (eds) (2002) *Consuming Health: The Commodification of Health Care*. London and New York: Routledge.

Henriksen, M. and Heyman, B. (1998) 'Values and health risks', in B. Heyman (ed.) *Risk, Health and Health Care: A Qualitative Approach*. London: Arnold.

Heyman, B. (ed.) (1998) *Risk, Health and Health Care: A Qualitative Approach*. London: Arnold.

Heyman, B. and Henriksen, M. (1998) 'Being old and pregnant', in B. Heyman (ed.) *Risk, Health and Health Care: A Qualitative Approach*. London: Arnold.

Jagose, A. (1996) *Queer Theory*. Melbourne: Melbourne University Press.

Joffe, H. (1999) *Risk and 'The Other'*. Cambridge: Cambridge University Press.

Larson, J.S. (1999) 'The conceptualization of health', *Medical Care Research and Review* 56(2): 123–36.

Lupton, D. (1995) *The Imperative of Health: Public Health and the Regulated Body*. London: Sage.

O'Malley, P. (2004) *Risk, Uncertainty and Government*. London: Glasshouse Press.

Petersen, A. (2005) 'The metaphors of risk: Biotechnology in the news' (Editorial introduction), *Health, Risk and Society* 7(3): 203–8.

Petersen, A. and Lupton, D. (1996) *The New Public Health: Health and Self in the Age of Risk*. London: Sage, and Sydney: Allen & Unwin.

Pidgeon, N., Kasperson, R.E. and Slovic, P. (eds) (2003) *Social Amplification of Risk*. Cambridge: Cambridge University Press.

Rose, N. (1990) *Governing the Soul: The Shaping of the Private Self*. London: Routledge.

Rose, N. (1999) *Powers of Freedom: Reframing Political Thought*. Cambridge: Cambridge University Press.

Skolbekken, J. (1995) 'The risk epidemic in medical journals', *Social Science and Medicine* 40(3): 291–305.

Slovic, P. (2000) *The Perception of Risk*. London: Earthscan.

Watney, S. (1997) *Policing Desire: Pornography, Aids and the Media* (third edn) London: Cassell.

Wilkinson, I. (1999) 'News media discourse and the state of public opinion on risk', *Risk Management: An International Journal* 1(4): 21–31.

Wilkinson, I. (2001) *Anxiety in a Risk Society*. London: Routledge.

Chapter 2

Unlimited medicalization? Risk and the pathologization of normality

John-Arne Skolbekken

In June 2003 professors Nick Wald and Malcolm Law launched their strategy to reduce cardiovascular disease by more than 80 per cent in an article in the BMJ (Wald and Law 2003). As such disease affects nearly half the population in many Western countries, the strategy would be a triumph for preventive medicine, provided its implementation were to match its estimated success. This bold aim is to be achieved by the creation of the Polypill, a pill combining six different ingredients known to be effective against the most important risk factors for cardiovascular disease. Besides being offered to people who have already developed cardiovascular disease, Wald and Law (2003) proposed that the Polypill should be taken daily by everyone aged 55 and above for the rest of their lives, regardless of their risk factor level.

In his Editor's Choice column Richard Smith described the articles by Wald, Law and colleagues as possibly the most important articles to be published in the BMJ for over 50 years (Smith 2003a). He also predicted that this breakthrough could lead to the future redundancy of cardiologists and cardiac surgeons. Luckily, this redundancy could be turned into another health care triumph, depending on the successful transformation of heart specialists into psychiatrists. Provided that the Polypill would be made available in supermarkets and pubs, without any diagnostic interventions by doctors, the strategy would also find its way around medicalization as no doctor need be involved.

Whether such comments represent euphoria or sheer irony is a matter of interpretation. It remains to be seen whether the Polypill strategy will come true or remain science fiction. What is of interest here is that it represents no major breach from recent developments within preventive medicine. It may simply be seen as the next logical step in a trend of including ever-increasing groups of symptom-free individuals in the realm of medicine.

An illustration of this has been given through the combination of data from the Nord-Trøndelag Health Study (HUNT 2) (see Holmen *et al.* 2003 for a closer description) and the 2003 European guidelines on cardiovascular disease prevention (DeBacker *et al.* 2003). The outcome of this pairing of data from one of the longest living populations in the world and the medical experts' guidelines for clinical practice is that half the 25-year-olds and 90 per cent of the 49-year-olds have blood cholesterol and blood pressure levels that place them above the guidelines' cut-off points for medical intervention. Implementation of the guidelines thus renders three out of four Norwegian adults in need of medical attention (Getz *et al.* 2004).

These interventions involve established diagnostic technologies such as blood pressure measurements and techniques for lifestyle change. As such there is little new in this compared to what has been described in earlier texts on the new public health and individuals' responsibility for their own health through self-regulatory behaviour (see Ogden 1995 and Petersen and Lupton 1996 for examples). What we witness is the medicalization of life, which has been going on for some time already. There have been developments over the past decade, however, that are worth noting. An escalation of the medicalization of life has taken place, through the pathologization of normality and the removal of the divide between preventive and clinical medicine. This latter change is demonstrated by the replacement of lifestyle changes by chemical prevention as the major mode of achieving the goals of preventive medicine.

About this chapter

The aim of this text is to present a critical analysis of recent developments. In doing so the emphasis will be on investigating how risk calculations within modern medicine are playing a central role in the ordering of reality. These calculations form the basis for a 'rationality for governing the conduct of individuals, collectivities and populations' (Dean 1999: 177). Within this frame of analysis risk is not seen as a realist entity, but as something that 'is a way of representing events in a certain form so they might be governable in particular ways, with particular techniques and for particular goals' (ibid.). The goal in question is nothing less than human well-being, which actors in society are trying to achieve through the management of life itself within the frame of what has been called risk politics (Rose 2001).

A central theme of this analysis is to investigate the close connection between risk calculation and medicalization. According to Conrad (1992: 209) 'medicalization describes a process by which nonmedical problems become defined and treated as medical problems, usually in terms of illnesses or disorders'. Within the calculated rationality of risk this process happens through the discursive transformation wherein normal body functions become risk factors that subsequently become diseases that demand medical attention. So, rather than observing a pattern wherein people experience symptoms that lead them to see their doctor, we are witnessing a process wherein research findings indicate that people without symptoms are in need of help. This leads doctors to actively target people who feel healthy through various screening programmes or case finding in general practice. Another characteristic of this medicalization process is the constant widening of the categories of symptom-free individuals in need of medical attention. Such expansions more often than not come subsequent to what is perceived as a successful medical intervention on the risk factor in question.

The analysis will be focused on the present risk discourse. As this discourse is clearly normative, the analysis will consequently also have normative elements. This normative aspect is based on scepticism about the uncritical presentation of possible positive outcomes of preventive medicine. As such it is partly situated within what has been called the medicalization critique (Lupton 1997). Central to this critique is that medicalization involves processes in which people are dominated through the practices of medical interventions that are at best useless or at worst directly harmful to people's health. Within this literature much attention has been given to the role of the medical profession; however, lately the pharmaceutical industry has also come to be seen as a central actor in the medicalization processes (Conrad 2005). In its most simplistic form the medicalization critique may be seen as an attempt at identifying a grand conspiracy within modern medicine. The ambition behind this text is to provide an analysis that also takes into consideration the critique of the medicalization hypothesis.

It is rather an attempt at showing how humans, armed with the power of scientific knowledge and a belief in their increased control over life and death, have created a situation whereby life in the modern world can be perceived as somewhat of a failure in need of constant medical attention.

Risk and surveillance

The medicalization of life is rooted in the development of surveillance medicine as the dominant form of medicine in the twentieth century (Armstrong 1983, 1995). Its cardinal feature is the targeting of everyone, as nobody is perfectly healthy through its gaze. We are all potentially sick or at risk of developing a disease and eventually dying.

These ideas have been central to preventive medicine since early in the twentieth century (Armstrong 1983). It has, however, taken on a new meaning in the second half of the century, through the identification of risk factors, a conceptual invention attributed to the Framingham study (Rockhill 2001). This has also become manifest through the risk epidemic, seen in the medical journals as a reflection of the rise in scientific knowledge about risk factors in the latter half of the twentieth century (Skolbekken 1995). In its original version this epidemic was shown as an increase from around 1000 articles about risk in the latter half of the 1960s to more than 80,000 two decades later. A follow-up showed that the epidemic has resulted in another quarter of a million articles in the last decade of the twentieth century (Skolbekken 2000).

Present preoccupation with risk within surveillance medicine is not only reflected in the rising number of 'risk-articles', but also in the paramount importance, if not omnipotence, attributed to risk in the present medical discourse. The quotations below serve as illustrations of this:

- 'risk...touches upon every single aspect of health and human welfare' (British Medical Association 1987).

- 'Life is a mixture of risks, what would a risk-free life be like? – life is a process of selecting a cause of death' (Lowell Levin). Aphorism of the month in *Journal of Epidemiology and Community Health* November 2005.
- '...life in developed countries at present almost inescapably entails long term exposure to major risk factors...' (Rodgers 2003).
- 'Communicating risk: The main work of doctors' (Smith 2003b).

Risk's importance is also reflected by the general acceptance in the social science literature of the risk discourse as one of the dominant discourses in this time and age. It is at the same time blurring the traditional dichotomy of health and illness, as well as reflecting complex and unclear notions of causality. This is illustrated in the challenges posed in the process of communicating what may look like causality at the epidemiological group level to uncertainty at the individual level (Skolbekken 1998; Hollnagel 1999; Olin Lauritzen and Sachs 2001; Rockhill 2001).

Another significant characteristic of risk is that it cannot be perceived directly through experiences of the lived body, it can only be mediated through risk measurements and calculations. A person's blood sugar, blood pressure or blood cholesterol level can only be revealed through the application of surveillance technology. The same is true for a person's bone mass, which if reduced beyond certain limits is considered to be a major risk factor for osteoporotic fractures. As a consequence, individuals cannot trust their own bodies and become dependent upon the medical profession for confirmations of their health status.

This implies that the risk discourse leaves us with a constant awareness of our vulnerability (Skolbekken 2000; Robertson 2001). This is the at-risk status, which leaves the individual in a state of being healthy and ill at the same time (Gifford 1986). It 'is to feel well, to be asymptomatic, yet always to be aware of the potential for becoming otherwise' (Scott *et al.* 2005: 1870). A consequence of this status achieved through the practice of surveillance medicine is a state of worry. This worry is not necessarily the result of the identification of risk, but comes as a result of the health surveillance itself. It may thus affect people not seen to be at risk as well as those at risk (Olin Lauritzen and Sachs 2001).

This presents us with a paradoxical situation. Whereas the rationale behind surveillance medicine is the protection against our unavoidable vulnerability as humans, it also creates a constant reminder of this vulnerability. It is against this background that criticism has been raised, claiming that preventive medicine based on epidemiological risk factor epidemiology has severe side effects (Førde 1998).

The pathologization of normality

The continuous construction and reconstruction of deviance and normality has played an important role in surveillance medicine. It has contributed to medicalization through the calculation of risk as deviance from the statistically normal. An illustration of this is to be found in the World Health Organization's guidelines on osteoporosis which defines it as a bone mass density that is 2.5 standard deviations or more below the mean bone mass density in a reference population (WHO Study Group 1994). Osteoporosis is similarly a condition that has been identified as a risk factor quite recently. This is illustrated by the number of articles found by the combination of the words 'osteoporosis' and 'risk' in searches in Medline. Until 1970 no matches were found and only 59 such articles had been published a decade later. Changes happened during the next two decades, however, and at present every third article about osteoporosis is also an article about risk (Skolbekken 2000).

Manifest osteoporosis is not lethal in itself, but has severely disabling and painful consequences with its fractures of the hip, vertebra and/or wrists as its most common consequences. Equally disabling consequences are caused by cardiovascular disease. Besides causing heart attacks and strokes, it is a major cause of death in the Western world. These manifest diseases have several common features. They are all characterized by a long period of latent development, a rather abrupt manifestation, and a complex causal background.

To reduce the incidence of these diseases is an important goal in preventive medicine. Through epidemiological studies researchers have identified risk factors associated with the diseases. Despite the complexity of the causality behind cardiovascular disease and manifest osteoporosis, risk factors such as hypercholesterolaemia, hypertension, type 2 diabetes and osteoporosis have been given central positions in the aetiology of these diseases. As a consequence, interventions aimed at reducing these risk factors have become central targets in current preventive medicine. This central position can be seen as a result of the fulfilment of three vital criteria – these factors are easily measured, their risk status can be calculated and they can be made subject to manipulation. They are thus prime targets for human control and therefore play an important role in risk politics.

It is in the transformation of physiological factors into risk factors that the pathologization of normality occurs. An essential feature of blood pressure, cholesterol, blood sugar and bone mass is that they all serve important functions in the human body. It is only when they reach certain levels that they are defined as risk factors and become potentially pathological and receive a status that makes them legitimate for medical intervention.

This status is a result of negotiations within scientific and clinical medicine, resulting in clinical guidelines. Just as in the case of osteoporosis, medical experts make decisions about arbitrary cut-off points, drawing the line between those who are in need of medical attention and those who are not. Development of such guidelines is a prime example of risk politics at the macro level. For risk politics to be successful it also needs to be transformed into micro politics, which is happening at the personal level of doctor–patient communication. As those in need of medical attention have no experiences that they perceive as symptoms, it then becomes the work of doctors to make sure that they are made aware of their needs.

As medical knowledge expands, the arbitrary cut-off points are renegotiated, with revised guidelines as the outcome. A characteristic feature of these guidelines is that they include an increasing number of the population among those in need of medical intervention. In the latest revision of the American guidelines on hypertension such negotiations resulted in the reconstruction of what had previously been defined as a normal blood pressure into prehypertension (Chobanian *et al.* 2003). As a consequence it has been estimated that 60 per cent of the US population are affected by prehypertension or hypertension (Wang and Wang 2004). A similar estimation from India found that 47 per cent and 35 per cent of the urban population fulfil the criteria of prehypertension and hypertension, respectively, leaving a mere 18 per cent of one of the largest populations in the world without need of medical intervention (Chockalingam *et al.* 2005).

Hypertension is not the only condition judged to have a pre-condition. The same is also true for type 2 diabetes, where another set of guidelines is covering prediabetes. In the 2003 revision of the guidelines of the American Diabetes Organization, the criteria for impaired fasting glycaemia was lowered, with an estimated growth in the number of people who fulfil the criteria in the middle-aged populations of urban India, urban China and the USA by 78, 135 and 193 per cent, respectively (Borch-Johnsen *et al.* 2004).

Turning back to Norway and the part of the HUNT study that included bone scans to identify possible risk of osteoporosis, it has also been demonstrated that more than two-thirds of the women over 70 years fulfil the WHO criteria for osteoporosis (Forsmo *et al.* 2005). This is because the criteria of what constitutes normal bone mass density are based upon a young reference population. Despite the vast number of individuals at risk only 1 per cent of these women will experience an osteoporotic fracture. This illustrates the problem of predictability related to current risk estimates. It remains a paradox that, whilst 90 per cent of the 50-year-olds are at risk of cardiovascular disease, the death rate for the same disease is around 45 per cent in the Norwegian population. Hence the prediction will be correct in about 50 per cent of the cases. In other words, the same prediction could be achieved by the flipping of a coin. This does not, however, have the same aura of controllability attached to it as risk calculations.

The age criteria suggested for the introduction of the Polypill may be seen as a consequence of such imperfect predictions. Acknowledging that the best predictors of risk are those factors that cannot be changed, such as age, sex and previous disease, Law and Wald (2002: 1574) conclude that 'age is the most important determinant of risk'.

In sum these examples illustrate that the pathologization of normality works in various ways. Starting off with the construction of the statistically deviant as pathological it has developed into defining the statistically normal as pathological. In doing so we are also faced with the pathologization of normal life in the modern world as well as the pathologization of the ageing process. So far as longevity can be seen as an achievement of the progress of humans, it is an intriguing paradox that ageing has become the major risk factor in the pursuit of further longevity.

Faced with these masses of people in need of medical intervention, the picture of our future looks pretty glum. There is hope, however, if we are to believe the recent triumphs achieved by preventive medicine.

The success of preventive medicine

Whereas risk for some time has played an important part in documenting the vulnerability of humans, it has recently also come to play an important part in proving the success of preventive medicine. The most important proof has come through the demonstration of risk reductions achieved by preventive efforts. These demonstrations have mainly been produced by randomized controlled trials (RCTs), recognized as the 'gold standard' of scientific medicine.

When the West of Scotland Coronary Prevention study was to be published a press release told the public that 'People with high cholesterol can rapidly reduce their risk of having a first-time heart-attack by 31 per cent and their risk of death by 22 per cent, by taking a widely prescribed drug called pravastatin sodium' (cited from Skolbekken 1998: 1956).

Similar success stories appear regularly in the media, making people aware of new triumphs or 'landmark studies', as they are appealingly labelled. In its tabloid format, these messages are personalized and aimed at the reflexive consumer as 'good news for *your heart*', illustrating the complementary privatization of risk reduction. The good news is often based on a drug's risk-reducing effect, as proven through a RCT. Taken literally these messages can be read as if the ultimate controllability is to be achieved as death soon will be made extinct.

Framed as science news stories, such news can also be interpreted as the pharmaceutical industry's way around the ban on direct-to-consumer advertisements for their prescription drugs; that is, in all countries except the USA and New Zealand where this kind of advertisement is allowed. This development does also imply a change in the role of what Petersen and Lupton (1996) called the healthy citizen, characterized by the individual's responsibility for his or her own health through their lifestyle choices. Whereas the risk discourse for a long time has appealed to the moral virtue of this responsible citizen, there is a twist aimed at the smart consumer. The appeal is no longer only aimed at a healthy lifestyle, but at a consumer aware of available products that can benefit his or her health.

A related feature is the offering of risk factor tests in newspapers and on various web sites, like that of the American Heart Association. Again the emphasis is on the smart consumer rather than the moral abiding citizen. In one such newspaper story readers were told that a computer program was now offered for free by the producers of the test to every physician in the country. The consumers were thereby urged to bring their doctors out of their state of ignorance if they were unable to offer the test to their patients. Such programs are now quite commonly used by doctors, serving as a reminder of their duty to offer risk measurements and a calculation of the patient's personal risk of dying in the coming decade.

Computer programs are not the only reminder doctors get. They are also regularly reminded of the success of chemical prevention, through the marketing efforts of the pharmaceutical industry. Such prevention is offered as well-documented examples of evidence-based medicine. This also illustrates the fiscal nature of the present success of preventive medicine. As the risk discourse has provided us all with the status of being potentially sick, in need of intervention, a new and vast market has been opened for the pharmaceutical industry. The nature of their products provides the industry with two major advantages compared to its competitors: they are well suited for testing in RCTs and it demands no major lifestyle change from the consumer/patient.

Not only is the entry of the pharmaceutical industry into the domain of preventive medicine based on the success of its risk-reducing products, it also contains a discourse undermining the existence of the healthy citizen. Risk-reducing drugs are offered as the effective solution where the efforts of the healthy citizen fail. If hypertension and hypercholesterolaemia are seen as risk factors created by a sedentary lifestyle, as well as wrongful diet and smoking, the pharmaceutical industry offers the perfect solution by means of effective prevention without changing behaviour. Health problems acquired by means of consumption through the mouth may thus be cured by the same mode of consumption. This is a point that has also been made clear for doctors through the pictures used for an antihypertensive drug (Malterud 2002), as well as in academic texts presenting the lifestyle efforts of lay people as failures (Wald and Law 2003). Chemical prevention is thus presented as a winner because it appears to offer better control.

Another conspicuous feature of the apparent success of preventive medicine is to be found in a selective use of risk information. In the vocabulary of epidemiology, risk reductions may be communicated both as relative risk reductions and as absolute risk reductions. The relative estimate is normally a much bigger figure than the absolute one, leaving an impression of a higher risk-reducing effect. This is illustrated by the press release presented above, where the numbers given are relative risk reductions. In terms of absolute risk reductions, the achieved effects could be stated as a 1.9 per cent reduction for first-time heart attacks and a 0.9 per cent reduction of deaths. Stated otherwise, people improved their chances of survival from 98.3 per cent to 98.8 per cent by taking the drug (Skolbekken 1998). The selective communication of relative risk reductions has proved profitable, as doctors and other decision makers are more inclined to prescribe drugs when faced with messages in this format compared to other formats. Not only has the strategy been used when addressing the medical profession, it has also been extensively used when risk reductions have been communicated through the mass media (Moynihan *et al.* 2000).

Judging by the sales numbers for drugs with a risk-reducing effect, this has been a successful communication strategy. The size of the success of chemical prevention remains somewhat of an enigma, however. This is in part related to the amount of uncertainty involved. Taking uncertainty into consideration, I was able to make the following statement based on the outcome of the West of Scotland Coronary Prevention study:

Medicine is not an exact science. Therefore, 200 men without any prior heart disease have to swallow 357,700 tablets over five years to save one of them from dying from coronary heart disease. This is due to the fact that no exact knowledge exists as to whom of these 200 will benefit from the treatment.

(Skolbekken 1998: 1957)

Rephrasing the message in this manner can be seen as a way of undermining the power of risk calculations and thus making them a less useful tool in the governing of human conduct. This illustrates that for risk to be a tool of governance it must be communicated in ways that emphasize control rather than uncertainty. In the current risk discourse governance is achieved through the presentation of group risk as individual risk, thereby disguising the uncertainty involved. As there are indications that patients' compliance is reduced the more informed they get, the success of preventive medicine can be seen as relying on the withholding of information about uncertainty. To tell the truth, the whole truth and nothing but the truth may therefore be a poor way of governance.

Medicalization and its limits

From what has been presented so far it is reasonable to conclude that there has been a continuous escalation of medicalization, involving the expansion of categories of the potentially ill over the last decades. When analysing the medicalization process it may be overly tempting to launch a conspiracy theory with two obvious culprits – the medical profession and the pharmaceutical industry. The medical profession has traditionally been seen as the powerful party towards whom the medicalization critique has been focused (Lupton 1997).

Without explicitly mentioning medicalization, Rose (2001) gives the pharmaceutical industry a prominent position in modern risk politics through its funding capacity within the life sciences. This view seems to be seconded by Conrad (2005) who notes that the pharmaceutical industry has played a more active part in the development of medicalization and portrays the industry as the new engine of medicalization. Further support for this claim is also given by Moynihan and Cassels (2005) who portray recent developments as a result of the pharmaceutical industry's efforts to sell sickness to the healthy population. The move away from lifestyle interventions towards chemical prevention described above is thus one of several observations of the connection between medicalization and the efforts of the pharmaceutical industry. In line with Rose's (2001) claim that risk politics makes life open to shaping and reshaping at the molecular level, preventive medicine is moving away from changing behaviour to changing cellular processes by means of chemical prevention.

To state that the escalation of medicalization is taking part because patients are being made victims of medicalization by doctors and their allies in the pharmaceutical industry would, however, be a mechanistic simplification. Taking as a starting point that recent developments are not just random events, it may prove fruitful to ask who it is that has an interest in an escalation of medicalization. In seeking the answer to this question we should look for the actors who support the goal of human well-being through the application of risk politics. This widens the number of possible suspects, as the prevention of premature deaths may be in the interest of public health authorities, health insurance companies, the mass media, politicians, lay people and patient organizations, as well as the mentioned profession and industry.

A way of expanding our understanding of medicalization would be to study the practices of these actors within the frame of risk politics through an interconnected set of analyses. At present many such studies can be found involving risk communication between doctors and patients. These studies can, however, only be properly understood against the background of other similar interactions, such as those between doctors and the pharmaceutical industry, in the format of drug advertisements or personal communication between doctors and sales representatives, and between the industry and the media, politicians or patient organizations, respectively. Rather than using Conrad's (2005) engine metaphor, a perhaps more useful metaphor is that of the pharmaceutical industry as the spider weaving a web of interactions upon which medicalization is based.

When studying such interactions, a likely discovery is that there are both common interests and conflicts of interest between these actors. These conflicts of interest also reflect a power struggle between the involved parties. An example of such a process was demonstrated by what in Norway came to be known as the Fosamax-case, after the name of a drug aiming at the reduction of osteoporotic fractures (Skolbekken 2001). At the knowledge level this was a conflict between a pharmaceutical company and the Norwegian health authorities over the interpretation of the results of a randomized controlled trial. On an economical level it was a conflict about who should pay the bill for chemical prevention of osteoporosis. Politically the conflict was about whether the provision of chemical prevention was to be seen as a feminist triumph or medicalization of women. Finally, on a moral level it was a question about defining the heroes and the villains in this conflict.

The development of the conflict was presented over a two-year period through nearly 40 articles in one of the largest national newspapers in Norway. A characteristic of the newspaper stories was that the pharmaceutical company started the process as heroes and ended up as villains. Despite losing the moral battle, they won the financial battle as their drug ended up on the blue prescription list, meaning that the national health insurance scheme is paying the majority of the prescription costs. Whether the outcome was a victory for feminism or another defeat at the hands of medicalization remains a matter of opinion. This also illustrates that what is going on is also a power struggle over the framing of the issue.

The Fosamax-case also illustrates that there are several modes of governance at work simultaneously. The blue prescription system is an example of social insurance whereby treatment is based on the solidarity principle; the economic risk is equally shared among the members of society. In the case of lifestyle diseases this solidarity also provides for those that fail to fulfil their personal responsibilities as healthy citizens. In the case of chemical prevention/treatment help is portrayed as contributed through a risk-reducing technology that has been developed within a liberal market economy.

An intriguing question that arises is how medicalization can happen if we know that it is bad for us and we know who is to blame for it. Indeed, if we know that the pharmaceutical industry is selling sickness, who is buying and why? Moynihan and Cassels' (2005) answer seems to be that people buy out of fear brought upon them by the pharmaceutical industry. If this is true, then medicalization may be seen as the outcome of irrational thoughts and behaviour.

Although fear and worry play a part, my claim would be that medicalization primarily is the outcome of the rational actions of major actors in modern society. In line with Dean's (1999) analysis the answer is to be found in the ordering of life constructed through risk calculation, which is rendering medical interventions into normal people's lives as most rational, backed by the best scientific evidence modern medicine can provide.

Part of the explanation behind the escalating medicalization is therefore to be found in the present discourse that makes it a duty for doctors to identify people at risk of cardiovascular disease and to offer them risk-reducing chemical prevention. Central to this discourse is that it is supported by science, thus making a refusal to fulfil the role obligations not only immoral, but also an act of irrational proportions in denial of scientific evidence.

Despite this there is considerable resistance against medicalization, which makes it possible to argue that there are limits to medicalization (Williams and Calnan 1996). One reason for such resistance is to be found in the existence of a lay epidemiology, reflecting the imprecise nature of epidemiological knowledge (Davison et al. 1991). Resistance among patients may come from many sources, and come to be explained in various ways. Whether what has traditionally been labelled non-compliance is an act of ignorance or the rational act of an empowered autonomous agent is open to debate.

Resistance to the present medicalization has also been offered from within the ranks of general practice. Based on the observation that current guidelines not only contribute to making the healthy into patients, but that they are also taking the medical profession's attention away from the really sick in favour of the healthy, current preventive practices have been claimed to be unethical (Hetlevik 2000). Such resistance is offered in opposition to the dominant position within the medical profession, mainly fronted by cardiologists. Central to this power struggle within the profession is the epistemological struggle over what represents the truth in scientific medicine, as well as the struggle over what identifies the good doctor.

The fact that the BMJ published a special issue (13 April 2002) on medicalization can also be seen as a form of resistance, reflecting a state of critical self-reflection within the medical profession. Whether such reflection will lead to changes in the practice of medicine remains to be seen. Current sales of drugs for hypertension, hypercholesterolaemia and osteoporosis indicate that medicalization is not suffering severe setbacks as a result of such reflections.

Existing guidelines and chemical prevention, including the Polypill, illustrate that there is a considerable potential for unlimited medicalization within the present discourse. Whether this potential will be realized or not depends on the outcome of several ongoing battles over what constitutes valid medical knowledge and how good medical practice is to be defined. These battles are literally about people's hearts and people's minds. The expansion of medicalization is due to the fact that it has a lot of appeal. It appeals to both the helper and the helped, and it can be backed by a scientific rationality as well as being a sound business. It is in line with the consumerist ethos as well as being framed within the rights of the citizen and the duties of civil society.

Concluding remarks

The present risk discourse represents a particular ordering of reality, providing a way of protection from and control over the vulnerability that we as humans are faced with. If what really is at stake here is people's lives, there should also be room for critical reflections about whose lives and whose vulnerability are excluded from the dominant discourse. As has been mentioned above, the morals of present risk politics may be questioned if it results in a reallocation of resources from the sick to the healthy.

On a larger scale this reallocation can already be seen to be taking place as the majority of medicines that are produced today are for the benefit of the lifestyles of the rich world, whereas lifesaving medicines for the poor are not available (Trouiller et al. 2001). A possible explanation for this is that the vulnerability of the poor fails to come into the realm of risk politics. Whereas the risk of poverty and its related miseries can be calculated, remedies are not to be found on the individual and molecular level. A major feature of current risk politics is thus that it provides for those that can pay rather than for the most vulnerable among us.

References

Armstrong, D. (1983) *The Political Anatomy of the Body: Medical Knowledge in Britain in the Twentieth Century.* Cambridge: Cambridge University Press.

Armstrong, D. (1995) 'The rise of surveillance medicine', *Sociology of Health and Illness* 17: 393–404.

Borch-Johnsen, K., Colagiuri, S., Balkau, B., Glumer, C., Carstensen, B., Ramachandran, A. *et al.* (2004) 'Creating a pandemic of prediabetes: The proposed new diagnostic criteria for impaired fasting glycaemia'. *Diabetologica* 47: 1396–402.

British Medical Association (1987) *Living with Risk.* Chichester: John Wiley and Sons.

Chobanian, A.V., Bakris, G.L., Black, H.R., Cushman, W.C., Green, L.A., Izzo, J.L. *et al.* (2003) 'The seventh report on the joint national committee on prevention, detection, evaluation, and treatment of high blood pressure: The JNC 7 report', *JAMA* 289: 2560–72.

Chockalingam, A., Ganesan, N., Venkatesan, S., Gnanavelu, G., Subramaniam, T., Jaganathan, V. *et al.* (2005) 'Patterns and predictors of prehypertension among "healthy" urban adults in India', *Angiology* 56: 557–63.

Conrad, P. (1992) 'Medicalization and social control', *Annual Review of Sociology* 18: 209–32.

Conrad, P. (2005) 'The shifting engines of medicalization', *Journal of Health and Social Behaviour* 46: 3–14.

Davison, C., Davey Smith, G. and Frankel, S. (1991) 'Lay epidemiology and the prevention paradox: The implication of coronary candidacy for health education', *Sociology of Health and Illness* 13: 1–19.

Dean, M. (1999) *Governmentality: Power and Rule in Modern Society.* London: Sage Publications.

DeBacker, G., Ambrosioni, E., Borch-Johnsen, K., Brotons, C., Cifkova, R., Dallongeville, J. *et al.* (2003) 'European guidelines on cardiovascular disease prevention in clinical practice', *European Heart Journal* 24: 1601–10.

Førde, O.H. (1998) 'Is imposing risk awareness cultural imperialism?', *Social Science and Medicine* 47: 1155–9.

Forsmo, S., Langhammer, A. and Forsen, L. (2005) 'Forearm bone mineral density in an unselected population of 2,779 men and women – The HUNT study, Norway', *Osteoporosis International* 16: 562–7.

Getz, L., Kirkengen, A.L., Hetlevik, I., Romundstad, S. and Sigurdsson, J.A. (2004) 'Ethical dilemmas arising from implementation of the European guidelines on cardiovascular disease prevention in clinical practice', *Scandinavian Journal of Primary Health Care* 22: 202–8.

Gifford, S.M. (1986) 'The meaning of lumps: A case study of the ambiguities of risk', in C.R. Janes, R. Stall and S.M. Gifford (eds) *Anthropology and Epidemiology: Interdisciplinary Approaches to the Study of Health and Disease.* New York: D. Reidel Publishing Co.

Hetlevik, I. (2000) 'Tilbake til de syke – forebygging på legekontoret i krise', in E. Swensen (ed.) *Diagnose Risiko.* Oslo: Universitetsforlaget.

Hollnagel, H. (1999) 'Explaining risk factors to patients during a general practice consultation: Conveying group-based epidemiological knowledge to individual patients', *Scandinavian Journal of Primary Health Care* 17(1): 3–5.

Holmen, J., Midthjell, K., Krüger, Ø., Langhammer, A., Holmen, T.L., Bratberg, G.H. *et al.* (2003) 'The Nord-Trøndelag Health Study 1995–97 (HUNT 2): Objectives, contents, methods and participation', *Norsk Epidemiologi* 13: 19–32.

Law, M.R. and Wald, N.J. (2002) 'Risk factor thresholds: Their existence under scrutiny', *BMJ* 324: 1570–6.

Lupton, D. (1997) 'Foucault and the medicalization critique', in A. Petersen and R. Bunton (eds) *Foucault, Health and Medicine.* London: Routledge.

Malterud, K. (2002) 'Når livsstil ikke nytter – medikamentell risikointervension for dårlige mennesker', in K.T. Elvbakken and P. Solvang (eds) *Helsebilder.* Bergen: Fagbokforlaget.

Moynihan, R. and Cassels, A. (2005) *Selling Sickness: How Drug Companies Are Turning Us All into Patients.* Crows Nest: Allen and Unwin.

Moynihan, R., Bero, L., Ross-Degnan, D., Henry, D., Lee, K., Watkins, J. *et al.* (2000) 'Coverage by the news media of the benefits and risks of medication', *New England Journal of Medicine* 342: 1645–50.

Ogden, J. (1995) 'Psychosocial theory and the creation of the risky self', *Social Science and Medicine* 40: 409–15.

Olin Lauritzen, S. and Sachs, L. (2001) 'Normality, risk and the future: Implicit communication of threat in health surveillance', *Sociology of Health and Illness* 23: 497–516.

Petersen, A. and Lupton, D. (1996) *The New Public Health: Health and Self in the Age of Risk*. London: Sage Publications.

Robertson, A. (2001) 'Biotechnology, political rationality and discourses of health risk', *Health* 5: 293–309.

Rockhill, B. (2001) 'The privatization of risk', *American Journal of Public Health* 91: 365–8.

Rodgers, A. (2003) 'A cure for cardiovascular disease?', *BMJ* 326: 1407–8.

Rose, N. (2001) 'The politics of life itself', *Theory, Culture & Society* 18: 1–30.

Scott, S., Prior, L., Wood, F. and Gray, J. (2005) 'Repositioning the patient: The implications of being "at risk"', *Social Science and Medicine* 60: 1869–79.

Skolbekken, J.-A. (1995) 'The risk epidemic in medical journals', *Social Science and Medicine* 40: 291–305.

Skolbekken, J.-A. (1998) 'Communicating the risk reduction achieved by cholesterol reducing drugs', *BMJ* 356: 1956–8.

Skolbekken, J.-A. (2000) 'Risiko for sykdom – vår tids epidemi?', in E. Swensen (ed.) *Diagnose risiko*. Oslo: Universitetsforlaget.

Skolbekken, J.-A. (2001) 'Risikoreduksjon på blå resept', in D. Thelle (ed.) *På den usikre siden: Risiko som forestilling, atferd og rettesnor*. Oslo: Cappelen Akademisk Forlag.

Smith, R. (2003a) 'The most important BMJ for 50 years?', *BMJ* 326 (7404).

Smith, R. (2003b) 'Communicating risk: The main work of doctors', *BMJ* 327 (7417).

Trouiller, P., Torreele, E., Olliaro, P., White, N. and Foster, S. (2001) 'Drugs for neglected diseases: A failure of the market and a public health failure?', *Tropical Medicine and International Health* 6: 945–51.

Wald, N.J. and Law, M.R. (2003) 'A strategy to reduce cardiovascular disease by more than 80%', *BMJ* 326: 1419–25.

Wang, Y.F. and Wang, O.J. (2004) 'The prevalence of prehypertension and hypertension among US adults according to the new Joint National Committee Guidelines', *Archives of Internal Medicine* 164: 2126–34.

WHO Study Group (1994) *Assessment of Fracture Risk and its Application to Screening for Postmenopausal Osteoporosis*. Geneva: WHO technical report series.

Williams, S.J. and Calnan, M. (1996) 'The "limits" of medicalization? Modern medicine and the lay populace in "late" modernity', *Social Science and Medicine* 42: 1609–20.

Chapter 3

Community care, risk and the shifting locus of danger and vulnerability in mental health

Joanne Warner

When read in relation to mental health care in post-asylum Britain, Mary Douglas' observation that 'the word *risk* now means danger; *high risk* means lots of danger' (1994: 24) has become almost axiomatic. However, questions of who or what is dangerous and who or what is vulnerable and in need of protection from harm have been central features of conflicting discourses on risk in mental health. At the time of writing, these conflicting discourses are clearly evident in the unresolved struggle in England and Wales over the reform or amendment of mental health legislation (Eastman 2006). The debate has centred largely on the supposed impact of the NHS and Community Care Act 1990 and an increasing 'conflation of violence with mental illness' (Pilgrim and Rogers 1999: 185). Following the closure of long-stay psychiatric hospitals there has been a focus in policy, the media and professional literature on a perceived increase in the risk of violence to others by people with a serious mental illness living in 'the community' (Department of Health 1998; Zito 1999). A particular preoccupation, especially in the media and among policy makers, has been the perceived increased risk of random acts of violence by mentally ill people against strangers in public places, as epitomised by the murder of Jonathan Zito by Christopher Clunis.[1] Concerns about such events have remained consistently high despite robust evidence to the contrary about the relative risks (see, for example, Shaw *et al.* 2004).

Following Clunis, the Department of Health stressed the importance of the removal of risk altogether:

> No patient should be discharged from hospital unless and until those taking the decision are satisfied that he can live safely in the community.
> (NHS Management Executive 1994: 1)

This zero tolerance approach to risk and emphasis on the concept of absolute safety was reflected in many subsequent policy documents but most powerfully in the Department of Health's 1998 white paper on mental health policy, *Modernising Mental Health Services*, which had as its subtitle *Safe, Sound and Supportive*. Underpinning this policy document was the assertion that community care policies had failed and that one of the main indicators of this failure was the presence of people with mental health problems in the community who were 'a danger to the public' (Department of Health 1998: 24). Community care policies themselves were thereby also declared 'unsafe'. The focus on those who may be a risk to others represented a shift away from the attention given to the 'scandals' of the 1960s and 70s which involved poor quality care for those considered vulnerable in large psychiatric institutions (Laurance 2003; Muijen 1996). Anxieties relating to 'the mad' have therefore shifted as the space they are perceived to occupy – both literal and symbolic – has changed (Leff 2001).

This chapter argues that the corollary of the construction of mental health service users as 'high-risk' to others has been the construction of 'the community' as vulnerable. The discourse of community as vulnerable is most readily discernible in mental health inquiries into homicides – made mandatory from 1994 by Virginia Bottomley as then Secretary of State for Health – and in the media accounts which invariably accompanied the events and then the publication of inquiry reports which followed them. The following quotation from one inquiry report illustrates the point:

> Winston Williams, a diagnosed schizophrenic with a history of violence and drug abuse...was allowed to roam the streets of Reading as a so-called 'care in the community' patient...My constituents wish to challenge the procedures which allowed Mr Williams to remain at large. (A Reading MP to the Home Secretary 24.05.00 and 19.09.00)
>
> (Johns et al. 2002: 3)

It is evident from this quotation that Williams was regarded as an outsider who had punctured the safety of a community of 'constituents'. The emphasis on his presence in public spaces such as the street is significant because of the sociocultural association this has with blurred boundaries and strangers as perplexing figures (Mossman 1997), as explored later in this chapter. It has been argued that policies have reconfigured the way professionals behave and are held accountable for their practice in relation to so-called 'high-risk' service users, and that the anxiety engendered by numerous homicide inquiry reports have been a powerful political tool in this respect (Eastman 1996; Muijen 1996; Szmukler 2000; Warner 2006). Further, there is evidence that the concept of dangerousness in the context of mental health is both gendered and racialised because it is young, black men who have been the focus of concern (Browne 1995; Keating et al. 2002; Sayce 1995) and this theme is explored in some depth.

The chapter also highlights the sociocultural significance of the mediating role that social work undertakes between mental health service users who are regarded as 'high-risk' and 'the community'. It draws on the accounts of 39 social workers to examine the concept of the 'high-risk' individual and also the interplay between discourses of risk, dangererousness and vulnerability in multidisciplinary professional practice with mental health service users. The chapter begins by examining the concept of vulnerability in the context of mental health in greater depth and then briefly considers the role of social workers under community care before outlining the empirical work that was undertaken.

The vulnerability/dangerousness axis in mental health

Vulnerability in a general sense has been defined as relating to 'the consequences of a perturbation, rather than its agent' (Downing and Bakker, quoted in Vatsa 2004: 10). People are therefore more or less vulnerable to the *effects* of disasters such as flooding – effects such as loss of life or home – rather than flooding itself. In relation to human services, this apparently straightforward distinction is more complex. According to government guidance on the protection of adults from abuse, a vulnerable adult is defined as anyone over eighteen years who:

> is, or may be, in need of community care services by reason of mental or other disability, age or illness; and who is or may be unable to take care of him or herself, or unable to protect him or herself against significant harm or exploitation.
>
> (Department of Health 2000: 9)

One of the residual impacts of post-asylum care policies is the continued construction of mentally ill people as a homogeneous group (Lewis *et al.* 1989: 181). Whilst there is little doubt that some individuals living with severe and enduring mental illness are in need of protection on a permanent basis due to their 'inherent vulnerability' (Kelly and McKenna 2004: 382), it is equally clear that not all mental health service users are, by definition, vulnerable and that vulnerability is dynamic over time rather than static. For some commentators, vulnerability can be more accurately understood as 'a way to describe the fragile and contingent nature of personhood' and, as such, we are all vulnerable in some sense (Beckett 2006: 3). The assumption of vulnerability among service users constructs the individual as dependent, passive and in need of intervention from services (Williams and Keating 2000: 33). It has connotations that are largely negative and suggests personal weakness rather than strength (Strehlow and Amos-Jones 1999: 261), underplaying the role that resilience and personal strategies to avert negative experiences often plays. However, when the dangers posed by mental health service users to *others* is emphasised in policy and practice, as already outlined, then the concept of vulnerability becomes even more problematic. Mental health service users are both *at* risk and perceived to be *a* risk to others and they thereby represent a perplexing 'juxtaposition of threat and vulnerability' (Moon 2000: 214).

Vulnerability in the context of mental health services is a central concept because it implies a lack of agency or responsibility which, in turn, places a responsibility on others to work with individuals at the margins, particularly professionals such as social workers, as emphasised by Douglas:

It seems that if a person has no place in the social system and is therefore a marginal being, all precaution against danger must come from others. He cannot help his abnormal situation. This is roughly how we regard marginal people in a secular, not a ritual context. Social workers in our society, concerned with the after-care of ex-prisoners, report a difficulty on resettling them in steady jobs, a difficulty which comes from society at large. A man who has spent any time 'inside' is put permanently 'outside' the ordinary social system...The same goes for persons who have entered institutions for the treatment of mental disease.

(2002: 121)

Significantly, when addressing the question of why community care is regarded as having failed, Leff (2001) pinpoints the symbolic significance of the 'architectural presence' of asylums and their replacement with more nebulous and dispersed forms of community care so that 'A good community psychiatric service is virtually invisible' (Leff 2001: 381). The increased visibility of mental health service users, particularly in urban inner-city areas (Moon 2000), means that everyday encounters of the mundane yet threatening kind described by Giddens are simply more frequent:

mental illness...reminds us of the fragility of the day-to-day conventions by which our experience both of social reality, and the basic parameters of existence more generally, is ordered...Goffman, rather than Foucault, may be right about mental illness: it represents an incapacity or an unwillingness to conform to some of the most basic 'situational proprieties' that everyday interaction presumes.

(1991: 205)

Such mundane threats to 'our' sense of well-being are powerful in the imagination, even in the absence of actual lived encounters with those who may be visibly mentally distressed. This is because of the wide dissemination of powerful narratives about the much more dramatic threat personified by Christopher Clunis. 'We' are all potentially vulnerable to this type of threat because the nature of the attack perpetrated by Clunis was random and happened in a public space. 'The community' has been newly reconstructed as vulnerable because the dividing line between 'us' and 'them' is perceived to be more porous than before and all strangers are potentially implicated.

It is therefore not surprising that mental health professionals are increasingly charged with the task of being seen, both literally *and* symbolically, to protect the community from harm. The constant attempts to revise the legal structure for mental health, the guidance to professionals and inquiries into their conduct, can all be regarded as attempts to impose new order on the subjective fears associated with mundane encounters and imagined threats as well as the 'real risks' that might arise from the conduct of embodied individuals. As Mossman (1997) has argued, debates that focus simply on 'factual refutations' of media distortions of the risks associated with mental illness and community care may well underestimate the culturally *symbolic* importance of such persistent narratives. The chapter now turns to consider the role of social work in community care.

'Working the social': social work, governmentality and community care

It has been argued that the shift from hospital-based mental health care to community care has involved a dispersal of disciplinary strategies in the Foucauldian sense (Cohen 1985). The same ideological positions that were witnessed in asylums – mainly in the form of medical dominance – have shifted to new and more dispersed sites, specifically the management in the community of the 'dangerous welfare "other"' (Ellis and Davis 2001: 138). Social workers, along with psychiatrists, are therefore at the front line in terms of public and political expectations about how the perceived risks associated with rapid social change in mental health care should be managed or 'policed'.

For Foucauldian theorists, governmentality in its contemporary form is characterised by neo-liberalism, an integral aspect of which is the role played by expert knowledge to survey the population, or the 'body' of society, and to ensure its productivity. Whilst this 'discipline' can take the form of explicit means of control, it is more closely identified with forms of regulation which are directed at individuals who come to police themselves. Lupton has provided a useful summary of how risk can be understood in the context of a governmental strategy:

> Risk is governed via a heterogeneous network of interactive actors, institutions, knowledges and practices. Information about diverse risks is collected and analysed...Through these never-ceasing efforts, risk is problematised, rendered calculable and governable. So, too, through these efforts, particular social groups or populations are identified as 'at risk' or 'high risk', requiring particular forms of knowledges and interventions.
>
> (1999: 87)

It has been argued that the shift to a focus on risk in social administration has profound implications for professional practice (Castel 1991). The chief characteristic of this shift is that intervention is now focused upon constellations of 'risk factors' rather than upon concrete individuals or groups of individuals, with the consequence that *'there is no longer a subject'* (1991: 288, emphasis in original). The shift to risk heralds a new approach to surveillance which Castel terms 'systematic predetection' (p.288) whereby risk assessment starts with a general definition of the dangers to be prevented rather than with the direct experience of some kind of threat based on contact with an individual. Castel identifies this shift, not only in professional practices within psychiatry but also in all of the social care professions, where increasing detachment from risky individuals is emphasised. Parton

(1996) has identified one such form of detachment in the virtual abandonment of 'relationship' in social work in favour of care packages, where monitoring is the core activity.

Whilst theorists such as Castel (1991) and Parton (1996) suggest that social work may have already lost the struggle to retain a focus on the subjectivity of service users rather than objective risk factors, Philp's (1979) historical perspective on social work predicts considerable areas of continuity rather than change in the way social work might be expected to operate under community care. This is because the space within which social work operates has always been *in between* objectified individuals and their subjectivity, and its role has historically been one of *mediation* between the two. Social work has thus been defined as a 'liminal profession' (Christie 2001: 12; Warner and Gabe 2004). According to Philp (1979), social work practice is defined by the following three operations: the creation of subjects, the integration of objective characteristics and the function of speaking for the subject. The operation of creating subjects is described as follows:

> The creation of subjects is essential to mediation. The social worker faced, on the one hand, with an objectified vandal and, on the other, with a legal discourse has to attempt to present the underlying subjectivity of the vandal... The social worker does not say that the vandal did what he [sic] wanted to do, for in so doing the role of the social worker would disappear. What he does, rather, is to allude to the underlying character, the hidden depths, the essential good, the authentic and the unalienated. In doing so he is producing a picture of the vandal as a subject who is not immediately visible but who exists as a possibility, a future social being. Even if he does this without hope or cynically, he does it because it is the major factor which differentiates him from the policeman, the lawyer, doctor or psychiatrist. The object that these discourses deal with is one which is constructed out of facts and objective utterances. With his place in and between these the social worker cannot help but try to create people, subjects, where everyone else is seeing cold, hard, objective facts.
>
> (Philp 1979: 99)

Philp points out that social work cannot defend the subjective status of all individuals, but is 'allocated those whose objective status is not too threatening' (p.99). Significantly, the boundaries that define those who are too threatening are constantly under negotiation. This chapter argues that a period of sustained and intense negotiation is underway in relation to the entire 'heterogeneous network of interactive actors, institutions, knowledges and practices' (Lupton 1999: 87) that form contemporary mental health services and that the twin concepts of dangerousness and vulnerability are at the centre of this network. The chapter explores these ideas in greater depth by drawing upon qualitative materials from an empirical study of risk work amongst mental health social workers, but first offers a description of the approach taken to data collection and analysis.

Methods

This chapter draws on data that were collected in an inner-city social services department in England in the mid to late 1990s. The research was funded jointly by the Economic and Social Research Council and the local authority concerned in the form of a collaborative research studentship. The aims of the project were to explore the processes involved in the assessment and management of risk by mental health professionals. Whilst the initial emphasis was on the evaluation of professional practice in relation to risk, the study evolved into one that engaged more with interpretive approaches and focused on the *meaning* of risk for professionals through the analysis of qualitative materials. The catchment area in which the research took place was socio-demographically diverse and the psychiatric morbidity of the population was high compared with the national average. Participants comprised all 39 social workers working for the department who were qualified as approved social workers[2] (ASWs) under the Mental Health Act 1983, including six team managers. The identities of participants and service users were protected by using a coding system to replace all names and by the use of pseudonyms for place names. These codes were applied throughout the process of transcribing and data entry. The research proposal was approved by the social services department and by the ethics committees of two mental health trusts.

Semi-structured interviews were carried out by the author with all 39 participants, each interview lasting approximately one and a half hours. With the consent of the participants, each interview was tape recorded. Each social worker also completed two questionnaires prior to their interview. Questionnaire 1 provided biographical information about them, for example the length of their experience as an approved social worker. Some details about each participant are given following each quotation in the chapter. Questionnaire 2 asked the social workers to identify service users on their caseload whom they would define as 'high-risk' and this yielded a second data set concerning 219 service users. A considerable amount of time during interviews was spent discussing the reasoning behind the definition of particular service users as 'high-risk'. Statements in the chapter concerning 'high-risk' service users refer to this population.

An initial analysis of the interview data was undertaken prior to the transcription of tapes so that general themes could be identified, in keeping with the need to become 'familiar with the data' (May 2001: 139). Once transcripts were available, the qualitative materials were coded by broadly following the three stages of open, axial and selective coding defined in Neuman's (1997) taxonomy (after Strauss 1987). The main objective in open coding was, as Berg puts it, to 'open inquiry widely' (2001: 251) with the aim of identifying themes in the shape of abstract concepts. The focus in axial coding was on organising key themes and ideas based on the initial set of 'open' codes. Finally, these themes were extended and reorganised so that patterns in the data could be elaborated. Miles and Huberman (1994) recommend the use of matrices and other cross-data display strategies in order to identify patterns, and these were also employed during the later stages of data analysis.

When people become hazards:
the 'high-risk' individual in mental health

It has been argued that the major difference between risks in human services and those in other contexts is that the main source of the potential threat or hazard in human services, particularly mental health services, is *people*: 'Recognising people as potential sources of hazard creates a number of tensions in human services that are difficult to resolve' (Alaszewski 2002: 185). This section explores some of these tensions in more detail and employs Hilgartner's notion of 'risk objects', whereby an entity is first defined as an object and then linked to harm (Hilgartner 1992). The strength of this approach is that any entity, including one that is wholly conceptual, can be considered a risk object.

In the present study, to be 'high-risk' in mental health was found to be increasingly synonymous with being a danger to other people rather than 'at risk' or vulnerable (such as through suicide or self-neglect). From the accounts of the six team managers, there was a consistent message about the political pressure to prioritise the management of risk of violence to others by service users over and above risks of self-harm, self-neglect or suicide. The following quote summarises the point:

Manager: '...I think it is very easy to just forget the people who are risks to themselves who aren't necessarily a risk to anyone else and it is easier to rate them at a lower risk generally...I suppose I feel the issue of risk is violence to others rather than to themselves.'

Interviewer: 'Do you have any ideas about why that is?'

Manager: 'I think that is part of a number of reasons, partly to do with, if you like, the kind of whole society type thing of the media, the inquiries and everything, which are very much focused on the injuries to other people, the murders of the public, injuries to the public, rather than the attention that is given to the numbers of mentally ill who commit suicide or commit serious self-harm. I think that is part of the human defensiveness part of our job, protecting society is probably higher than protecting the individual from themselves.'

(Interview 34, female manager with 7 years' ASW experience)

Such a statement illustrates the argument that risk in mental health has been politicised in explicit ways since the implementation of community care policies, with risk now meaning 'danger to others'. Within the network of risk and vulnerability constructed out of community care policies, mentally ill people have become 'risk objects' because of the perception that networks of containment (formerly in the shape of the asylum) under community care have failed. Social workers identify themselves as being held responsible for the management of 'new risks' and, in particular, for the wider role of 'protecting society'.

This is another example of the way social work practice has been reconstituted under community care, as illustrated by this respondent:

> I think there are big question marks about whether or not it is my job to manage risks if a client is not on any sort of order of the Mental Health Act; they don't want to see me; I have got my mandate for seeing them is pretty much non-existent, then I am sort of doubtful whether or not [I should]. There is something that smacks of 'Well, dump it all on the Care Managers, the ASW. It is their job to manage every risk of every client in the community.' And there is something that backs away from me of doing that because I can't do it, no one can do it. I can try within the confines of practice and the law to look at issues of risk with clients and do something...
>
> (Interview 14, female with 3 years' ASW experience)

Even though a number of new risk objects have been emplaced under community care policies, there have indeed been struggles over this process. As the social worker quoted above makes clear, the role assigned to them of managing 'every risk of every client in the community' is not one they have all readily accepted. It is clearly identified as being at odds with other aspects of their role. The next social worker quoted makes it clear that the perception of their new responsibilities under community care is one which the senior management of the local authority has felt obliged to endorse. He describes how press reports of an impending crisis led to the establishment of new care management (social work) posts, but that this simply reinforced the message that it was social workers who were responsible for managing all risks in the community:

> For example, last year we got extra care management posts after it was reported in the local paper that there will be 'Bedlam in the Streets'. A report from the Director that said he wanted to make sure that we carried out our responsibilities adequately...adequate services and reducing risk. The message was that there could be dangerous people on the streets, harming the public; clear implication that care managers were supposed to be doing that particular job.
>
> (Interview 2, male with 9 years' ASW experience)

The reference to 'the street' in this quote is an important one, as it illustrates how 'the street' has become a risk object linked to the potential for harm by someone with a mental health problem. The street has become a major site in which social workers perceive themselves as having taken on a particular set of new responsibilities under community care.

Risk was also identified closely with specific characteristics relating to age, 'race' and ethnicity and gender, such that young black men with a diagnosis of schizophrenia were a particular focus. This finding is consistent with findings in the literature that black men are more likely to be *perceived* as 'dangerous individuals' than people from other groups (Browne 1995; Dutt and Ferns 1998; Hollander 2001; Keating *et al.* 2002; Loring and Powell 1988). Homicide inquiry reports, exemplified by the inquiry into the murder of Jonathan Zito by Christopher Clunis, together with the powerful media accounts which have accompanied them, appear to have provided a template for this construction of risk (Neal 1998). This is illustrated by the following interview extract and the reference to the service user (who is an African Caribbean man in his thirties with a diagnosis of paranoid schizophrenia) as being a 'Christopher Clunisey type figure':

> He has actually got a history of violence; he doesn't like women; he has allegedly, *allegedly* I say because it was never brought to court, assaulted a 14-year-old girl; and he doesn't appear to consider that he has any problems at all so I consider him a high risk and in a way he is not going to have any support networks apart from us and the psychiatric team when he is outside of hospital because he has not done anything yet and I have a horrible feeling that he will, and all we can do is keep a very close eye on him. I do see him as a very Christopher Clunisey type figure; that he moves around London a lot and we have to continue to chase him, so I would say he was very, very high risk actually, when I think about it, because he won't have any support networks.
>
> (Interview 39, female manager with 8 years' ASW experience)

Similar themes about 'race' and the risk of violence emerged in a number of other interviews. The extract below exemplifies Prins' observation, following his investigation and report in 1993 into the death of Orville Blackwood in Broadmoor Hospital, that 'There was also a tendency to see such black patients as "big, black and dangerous" because of their size and ethnic origins, where there was no evidence for such an assumption' (1999: 132). The extract also has the additional feature of risks associated with sexualised behaviour and the man's ethnicity:

Interviewer: 'Were the risks perceived to be to himself or to others?'

ASW: 'Both. Part of this behaviour pattern was making inappropriate approaches to members of the opposite sex.'

Interviewer: 'Did that ever extend to actual contact physically as far as you know?'

ASW: 'As far as I know it didn't go as far as rape or anything like that, but he is a big built Afro-Caribbean man who would present as immediately threatening in any kind of approach and it was done in a very unsophisticated way.'

Interviewer: 'Where would you rank him [on your high-risk list]?'

ASW: 'We are struggling with this. At one end of the spectrum people will define him as a Christopher Clunis.'

(Interview 33, male with 4 years' ASW experience)

As Sayce (1995) has argued, the racist assumption that black men are more likely to commit rape or sexual assault has a longstanding history and it is this assumption, among others, which has prefigured the assumed link between violence, 'race' and mental illness. In this sense, young black men with schizophrenia have become 'significant actors' who are linked to harm in community care. Their *vulnerability*, in contrast, is rendered largely invisible. In the next section the chapter moves on to consider the location of risk in a wider context. This is most readily demonstrated by focusing on the theme of disagreement within multidisciplinary teams, which was one focus in the interviews with social workers.

Social work, psychiatry and the creation of vulnerable subjects

It has long been argued that one of the key issues in collaboration between psychiatrists and social workers is the important ideological difference between them in terms of the models of explanation applied to mental health/illness. In crude terms, psychiatry has been identified with medical models and social work with social models of explanation (Miller *et al.* 2001). These ideological differences are believed to be a major source of some of the divisions and conflicts which are said to occur within multidisciplinary teams and such differences were evident in some, although not all, of the interviews with social workers in the present study.

Analysis of the qualitative material from the present study showed that professionals working in multidisciplinary teams often interpreted the same information about risk differently, assessing the level of risk to be higher or lower than colleagues according to the different meanings they gave to it. The following extended extract serves to illustrate the complex ways in which these differences are related to ideological differences and the way risk and vulnerability are accordingly constructed by professionals:

Interviewer: 'Do you think that the psychiatrist normally shares your views about the level of risk faced or posed by this client?'

ASW: 'I think [the consultant psychiatrist] sees him as being higher risk than I would. I would definitely say that he has potential for doing serious damage to someone and [the consultant] has written a report that says she sees him as potentially committing homicide, which I would agree with certainly. However, the majority of the time I wouldn't particularly see [the service user] as being a risk, although I think [the consultant's] feelings are that he is potentially more of a risk more of the time.' [...]

Interviewer: 'Have there ever been any decisions taken in relation to the care of this client with which you have disagreed?'

ASW: 'Not really. I am saying that because I can see both sides. For example, I suppose [the service user] attending a day hospital, I can understand why both [the community psychiatric nurse and the consultant] think he should do that because he is obviously going to be in closer contact with services and he is going to be monitored more closely than he is doing so now on discharge. Whereas I can also see his point of view, which is that he doesn't actually see himself as fitting neatly into the mental systems...a lot of people he knows have attended there for quite a long time, are actually quite different in their level of functioning. He has had a very high level of independence and he wants to retain that. I think he is going quite a long way along the lines of how we want to work with him in terms of keeping in contact with us and I think expecting him to go to a day hospital five days a week would probably be counter productive [...] [the service user] does want to retain as much independence as he can but he recognises that he has had a couple of very severe breakdowns and he recognises that he needs to remain on medication if he is going to be reasonably sure of being stable...at least, I think he does... [...] OK, I am sure that he will have problems that he will have to face when in the community and I am fairly confident that he will be able to deal with a lot of these problems. I just feel that I can completely understand why he wants as normal a life as possible and, to me, I feel we should be supporting that more with clients rather than getting them to fit with our medical model.'

(Interview 7, male with 1 year's ASW experience)

It is important to note that the social worker quoted above constructs the day hospital as conceptually linked to harm by virtue of seeing this service user's attendance against his wishes as 'potentially counter productive' and putting him 'at risk'. From the social worker's account, the medical team view the attendance of this person at the day hospital solely as an effective means through which he can be monitored and the risk he *poses* thereby reduced. They have located risk in the person, identifying him as the very *embodiment* of risk in terms of a propensity for violence which is regarded as a permanent feature of his character. The alternative would be to see dangerousness as arising out of certain *circumstances* or conditions (Chiswick 1995). The social worker, in contrast, appears to regard this service user as vulnerable to the iatrogenic effects of the medical monitoring he is subject to as well as considering him 'a risk' to others and attempts to balance the two. Philp's (1979) notion of social work as engaging in the process of creating a subject and speaking for him is clearly evident here.

A similar pattern can also be seen in the following extract from another social worker from the same team, again with reference to disagreement with a psychiatrist. In this case, the focus is on medication as being linked with harm, but also 'hospital' which is constructed bi-dimensionally and therefore becomes a risk object because of the disruption caused by frequent admissions:

Interviewer: 'In your experience, are there any specific issues over which there are more likely to be disagreements with other professionals?'

ASW: 'I think there is always the issue of medicine and how people...what it means for someone to be taking medicine, and something else that is also very, very underplayed is the impact of someone's home. [Service user's name] last year was admitted to hospital three times, which [the consultant psychiatrist] interpreted as being a case that was poorly managed, inadequate medication, it was quite blaming what she was doing and she missed out that [the service user] was decamped from her flat because the flat was going to be renovated, moved to another place and then had to move back within that year as well and that completely shook her world and she broke down because she was so angry that these changes were being imposed on her and it wasn't helpful for [the consultant psychiatrist] to say: "Look at you, you just keep breaking down", blaming her, kind of thing, without understanding what was happening in her life and I think that is where I end up doing the most kind of advocacy work, by saying to medical people that, when you see someone who is two stone heavier than they were three months ago: "Look, what is their motivation for taking medicine? We are not offering them something that is helpful."'

(Interview 6, female with 6 years' ASW experience)

The medical team are portrayed as viewing the hospital admission and medication one-dimensionally as part of a risk management strategy, whilst the social worker views them as bi- or even multidimensional, since they each may also serve to *increase* the level of risk. Again, the vulnerability of the service user is emphasised in the social worker's account and in her attempt to mediate between psychiatrist and service user. It is *not* being argued here that the operation of creating subjects precludes social work from also engaging in processes of surveillance and control along with psychiatrists. The point is that social work can be understood as doing *both* by virtue of its role in speaking for others (Philp 1979).

Conclusions

This chapter has argued that mental health service users have been increasingly regarded as representing 'a risk' to others rather than being 'at risk' and vulnerable. This portrayal of them has been a central feature, not only of media coverage on the issue but also policy developments. It has been argued that the corollary of this construction of mental health service users is the construction of 'the community' as vulnerable in that it is portrayed as being at risk from random attacks by strangers with mental illness. The chapter has shown how the role of social work under community care has been to act as mediator between communities which have been newly cast as vulnerable and mental health service users who are often perceived as an homogeneous and threatening group. Social workers in the present study therefore perceived themselves as taking up a position 'in-between' individual service users and a fearful community. Further, they have been seen to engage in a process whereby the individual biographies of service users are brought to the fore, thus creating subjects rather than constellations of risk factors. The process of creating subjects also involves attempts to construct service users as vulnerable in the sense that they are exposed to harm. This process appeared to set social workers apart from their colleagues in the multidisciplinary team, forming the basis for disagreement between them. However, it has also been seen that this process has not precluded social workers from engaging in surveillance and control.

The fact that mental health professionals such as social workers appear to equate the concept 'high-risk' more readily with violence to other people than with behaviours more obviously associated with vulnerability such as self-harm or self-neglect raises complex and difficult questions concerning the moral equivalency of harmful outcomes. Outside the context of mental health services, it may be possible to argue that self-harm and harm to others are *not* moral equivalents. Fairburn (1995) has, to some extent, explored the philosophical question of the distinction between suicide and murder in this regard. But *within* mental health services, the moral questions are even more complex, given that mental health professionals owe a duty of care to service users in relation to *all* dimensions of risk and vulnerability, at least theoretically. This duty of care is expressed in mental health policy, guidance and legislation, such as policies relating to the reduction of the suicide rate, although, as shown in earlier discussions, this dimension of risk has received far less attention since the 1990s. A more robust re-articulation of the duty of care owed by professionals (and, de facto, owed by society at large) to mental health service users is needed to redress the balance which, for the time being at least, appears to have been lost.

The significance of the homicide inquiry into Christopher Clunis and the sense that he can be considered the archetypal 'high-risk' figure in mental health services appears to be endorsed by the social workers in the present study. It is clear that Clunis has had a profound impact on the way mental health professionals perceive some service users. The role that deep-rooted cultural fears may play, and the significance of 'race' in this respect, has been explored in this chapter. It has been argued that the 'mad stranger' has become a racialised and gendered category whereby young black men have come to embody the category high-risk in community care, regardless of their history of violence. The consequences of such racialised constructions of risk in terms of the lived experience of individual service users are profound: 'To be young and black, particularly for males, is to be deemed a greater risk and in need of increased surveillance and greater control...we are seen as requiring control as opposed to care...' (Browne 1995: 67).

There is therefore a strong sense in which racial otherness and embodiment, specifically in terms of the symbolic significance of 'black' (Shilling and Mellor 2001), have become central to contemporary constructions of risk in mental health, including in professional practice. In contrast, conceptualisations of young black men as vulnerable are largely absent, despite the overwhelming evidence of the risks they face – not least from within mental health services (Blofeld *et al.* 2003). The idea that the negative stereotyping of young black men is a reshaping of a much older stereotypical image is highly plausible. Hall *et al.*'s (1978) study of 'mugging' applied Cohen's (1973) seminal work about folk devils and moral panics to demonstrate how young black men are presented in the media as being prone to gratuitous violence against 'innocent' citizens on the streets.

The developments described in this chapter and by other commentators in the mental health field call for creative responses from practitioners and policy makers alike. There is clearly a need for the articulation of alternative visions of mental health and community care which can challenge the current orientation of policies, legislation and practice. To a great extent, the Mental Health Alliance has been one such development. This consortium of virtually all major mental health organisations, 78 in total, was formed in 1999 and has developed its own policy agenda (Mental Health Alliance 2005). New alliances are needed between and within service user movements and groups of practitioners if the bland statements contained within occupational standards and the 'shared capabilities' for mental health professionals, particularly those which concern challenging inequality, are to recover their meaning.

Notes

1 Christopher Clunis is a young African Caribbean man with a history of mental illness, who killed Jonathan Zito at Finsbury Park underground station in London in December 1992.
2 Approved social workers are mental health specialists who, together with psychiatrists, have legal powers to compulsorily detain people in hospital.

Acknowledgments

The author would like to thank the following: Professors Jonathan Gabe and Mike Bury for their valuable contributions to the ideas in this chapter; the Economic and Social Research Council, which funded part of the research; and everyone from the social services department where the research took place.

References

Alaszewski, A. (2002) 'Risk and dangerousness', in B. Bytheway, V. Bacigalupo, J. Bornat, J. Johnson and S. Spurr (eds) *Understanding Care, Welfare and Community: A Reader.* London: RKP.

Beckett, A.E. (2006) *Citizenship and Vulnerability: Disability and Issues of Social and Political Engagement.* Hampshire: Palgrave Macmillan.

Berg, B.L. (2001) *Qualitative Research Methods for the Social Sciences* (fourth edn). Boston: Allyn and Bacon.

Blofeld, J., Sallah, D., Sashidharan, S., Stone, R. and Struthers, J. (2003) *Independent Inquiry into the Death of David Bennett*, Norfolk, Suffolk and Cambridgeshire Strategic Health Authority.

Browne, D. (1995) 'Sectioning: The black experience', in S. Fernando (ed.) *Mental Health in a Multi-ethnic Society.* London: Routledge.

Castel, R. (1991) 'From dangerousness to risk', in G. Burchell, C. Gordon and P. Miller (eds) *The Foucault Effect: Studies in Governmentality.* London: Harvester Wheatsheaf.

Chiswick, D. (1995) 'Dangerousness', in D. Chiswick and R. Cope (eds) *Seminars in Practical Forensic Psychiatry.* London: Gaskell.

Christie, A. (2001) 'Gendered discourses of welfare, men and social work', in A. Christie (ed.) *Men and Social Work: Theories and Practices.* Hampshire: Palgrave.

Cohen, S. (1973) *Folk Devils and Moral Panics.* St Albans: Paladin.

Cohen, S. (1985) *Visions of Social Control.* Cambridge: Polity.

Department of Health (1998) *Modernising Mental Health Services: Safe, Sound and Supportive.* London: Department of Health.

Department of Health (2000) *No Secrets: Guidance on Developing and Implementing Multi-agency Policies and Procedures to Protect Vulnerable Adults from Abuse.* London: The Stationery Office.

Douglas, M. (1994) *Risk and Blame: Essays in Cultural Theory.* London: Routledge.

Douglas, M. (2002) *Purity and Danger.* London: Routledge Classics.

Dutt, R. and Ferns, P. (1998) *Letting Through Light: A Training Pack on Black People and Mental Health.* London: Department of Health.

Eastman, N. (1996) 'Towards an audit of inquiries', in J. Peay (ed.) *Inquiries after Homicide.* London: Duckworth.

Eastman, N. (2006) 'Reforming mental health law in England and Wales. The government's recent climbdown is not a victory: The real battle is about to begin', *British Medical Journal* 332: 737–8.

Ellis, K. and Davis, A. (2001) 'Managing the body: Competing approaches to risk assessment in community care', in R. Edwards and J. Glover (eds) *Risk and Citizenship.* London: Routledge.

Fairburn, G.J. (1995) *Contemplating Suicide: The Language and Ethics of Self Harm.* London: Routledge.

Giddens, A. (1991) *Modernity and Self-Identity: Self and Society in the Late Modern Age.* Cambridge: Polity Press.

Hall, S., Critcher, C., Jefferson, T., Clarke, J. and Roberts, B. (1978) *Policing the Crisis: Mugging, the State and Law and Order.* London: Macmillan.

Hilgartner, S. (1992) 'The social construction of risk objects: Or, how to pry open networks of risk', in J.F. Short and L. Clarke (eds) *Organizations, Uncertainties and Risk* (pp. 39–53). Boulder, CO: Westview Press.

Hollander, J.A. (2001) 'Vulnerability and dangerousness: The construction of gender through conversation about violence', *Gender and Society* 15(1): 83–109.

Johns, G., Sheppard, D. and Bowden, P. (2002) *Independent Inquiry into the Care and Treatment of Winston Williams.* Berkshire: Berkshire Health Authority.

Keating, F., Robertson, D., McCulloch, A. and Francis, E. (2002) *Breaking the Circles of Fear: A Review of the Relationship Between Mental Health Services and African and Caribbean Communities.* London: The Sainsbury Centre for Mental Health.

Kelly, S. and McKenna, H.P. (2004) 'Risks to mental health patients discharged into the community', *Health, Risk and Society* 6(4): 377–85.

Laurance, J. (2003) *Pure Madness: How Fear Drives the Mental Health System.* London: Routledge.

Leff, J. (2001) 'Why is care in the community perceived as a failure?', *British Journal of Psychiatry* 179: 381–3.

Lewis, D.A., Shadish, W.R., Jr. and Lurigio, A.J. (1989) 'Policies of inclusion and the mentally ill: Long-term care in a new environment', *Journal of Social Issues* 45(3): 173–86.

Loring, M. and Powell, B. (1988) 'Gender, race, and DSM-III: A study of the objectivity of psychiatric diagnostic behaviour', *Journal of Health and Social Behaviour* 29: 1–22.

Lupton, D. (1999) *Risk.* London: Routledge.

May, T. (2001) *Social Research: Issues, Methods and Process* (third edn). Buckingham: Open University Press.

Mental Health Alliance (2005) *Towards a Better Mental Health Act: The Mental Health Alliance Policy Agenda.* Available at: http://www.mentalhealthalliance.org.uk/policy/documents/AGENDA2.pdf (accessed July 2007).

Miles, M.B. and Huberman, A.M. (1994) *Qualitative Data Analysis: An Expanded Sourcebook.* California: Sage.

Miller, C., Freeman, M. and Ross, N. (2001) *Interprofessional Practice in Health and Social Care: Challenging the Shared Learning Agenda.* London: Arnold.

Moon, G. (2000) 'Risk and protection: The discourse of confinement in contemporary mental health policy', *Health and Place* 6: 239–50.

Mossman, D. (1997) 'Deinstitutionalization, homelessness, and the myth of psychiatric abandonment: A structural anthropology perspective', *Social Science and Medicine* 44(1): 71–83.

Muijen, M. (1996) 'Scare in the community: Britain in moral panic', in T. Heller, J. Reynolds, R. Gomm, R. Muston and S. Pattison (eds) *Mental Health Matters: A Reader.* London: Macmillan.

Neal, S. (1998) 'Embodying black madness, embodying white femininity: Populist (re)presentations and public policy – the case of Christopher Clunis and Jayne Zito', *Sociological Research Online* 3(4). Available at: http://www.socresonline.org.uk/3/4/2.html (accessed July 2007).

Neuman, W.L. (1997) *Social Research Methods: Qualitative and Quantitative Approaches* (third edn). Needham Heights: Allyn and Bacon.

NHS Management Executive (1994) *Guidance on the Discharge of Mentally Disordered People and their Continuing Care in the Community, HSG (94)27.* London: Department of Health.

Parton, N. (1996) 'Social work, risk and "the blaming system"', in N. Parton (ed.) *Social Theory, Social Change and Social Work.* London: Routledge.

Philp, M. (1979) 'Notes on the form of knowledge in social work', *Sociological Review* 27(1): 83–111.

Pilgrim, D. and Rogers, A. (1999) *A Sociology of Mental Health and Illness* (second edn). Buckingham: Open University Press.

Prins, H. (1999) *Will They do it Again? Risk Assessment and Management in Criminal Justice Psychiatry.* London: Routledge.

Sayce, L. (1995) 'Response to violence: A framework for fair treatment', in J. Crichton (ed.) *Psychiatric Patient Violence: Risk and Response.* London: Duckworth.

Shaw, J., Amos, T., Hunt, I.M., Flynn, S., Turnbull, P. and Kapur, N. (2004) 'Mental illness in people who kill strangers: Longitudinal study and national clinical survey', *British Medical Journal* 328: 734–7.

Shilling, C. and Mellor, P. (2001) *The Sociological Ambition.* London: Sage.

Strauss, A. (1987) *Qualitative Analysis for Social Scientists.* New York: Cambridge University Press.

Strehlow, A. and Amos-Jones, T. (1999) 'The homeless as a vulnerable population', *Nursing Clinics of North America* 34(2): 261–74.

Szmukler, G. (2000) 'Homicide inquiries: What sense do they make?', *British Journal of Psychiatry* 24: 6–10.

Vatsa, K.S. (2004) 'Risk, vulnerability, and asset-based approach to disaster risk management', *International Journal of Sociology and Social Policy* 224(10/11): 1–48.

Warner, J. (2006) 'Inquiry reports as active texts and their function in relation to professional practice in mental health', *Health, Risk and Society* 8(3): 223–37.

Warner, J. and Gabe, J. (2004) 'Risk and liminality in mental health social work', *Health, Risk and Society* 6(4): 387–99.

Williams, J. and Keating, F. (2000) 'Abuse in mental health services: Some theoretical considerations', *Journal of Adult Protection* 2(3): 32–9.

Zito, J. (1999) 'Community care: Past failures, future directions', *Probation Journal* 46(2): 101–5.

Chapter 4

Governmentality and the subpolitics of teenage sexual risk behaviour

Joost Van Loon

This chapter critically explores a particular theoretical perspective within risk research, namely that of 'governmentality' (Lupton 1999). This perspective, originally associated with the work of Foucault (1977, 1979, 1980) explores risks from the point of view of their functioning within systems of regulation and control, particularly those of the modern state (Burchell *et al.* 1991).[1] It suggests that risks enable forms of governing populations by providing legitimacy to both obtaining information (surveillance) of, as well as providing pervasive intervention (discipline) into, the everyday lives of people by state authorities.

It can be argued that Foucault's concept of governmentality lacks a sense of agency and motivation; that is, it does not tell us who drives this shift in governing people and why this became the preferred means to govern. There remains a suggestion that governmentality emerged simply because it was more effective and functional. However, the very fact that governmentality requires legitimation suggests that there is a political underpinning. This chapter argues that this legitimacy is derived from what Ulrich Beck (1997) has referred to as 'subpolitics'. That is, it is enabled by a form of politics that operates outside the realm of formal democratic procedures, but instead through expertise and lobbying (including demonstrations, direct action and other forms of extra-parliamentary political participation of, for example, social movements).

To substantiate this, I will draw upon the discourse of teenage sexual risk behaviour in the UK which has been deployed by the British government in its 'Teenage Pregnancy Strategy' (TPS). Exploring the basic premises of this strategy enables us to see how particular 'relations of risk-definition' (Beck 2000) have emerged as key elements of the way in which teenage sexuality is being governed. We will see how this discourse renders young people 'vulnerable' to the extent that their integrity as subjects is overruled by the need for pervasive control and regulation. It will also be shown that this discursive rendering is rooted in the subpolitical re-engineering of sexuality by means of (a) the growing importance of technoscientific expertise to visualize risks associated with teenage sexuality, (b) a shift in importance from primary socialization (within the family) to institutionalization (e.g. through schools) to anchor the significance of these risks, and (c) a translation of risks into costs and benefits that can be exchanged on markets and thereby given economic value (commodification). This enables us to widen the concept of subpolitics from Beck's original focus on pressure groups and social movements, to a host of apparently non-political agents, such as scientific experts, governance and commerce. This extension also entails a significant modification of the governmentality perspective on risk; rather than primarily government-based, we can see how governmentality entails an *ethos* that is pervasive throughout all aspects of modern life.

However, one issue that throws significant doubt on the efficacy of governmentality (and perhaps the lack of attention it pays to subversive strategies of avoiding surveillance and discipline of sexual behaviour by young people) is the fact that in the case of the TPS there is no tangible evidence of any success in the UK. Teenage pregnancies have only been reduced by a small percentage, yet simultaneously other indicators of teenage sexual risk behaviour, such as sexually transmitted infections (STIs), suggest that the strategy is failing as the rates of STI infections amongst young people continue to rise (Nicoll *et al.* 1999). Yet, despite lack of evidence of success, the TPS is not being reconsidered or modified. We need to ask why this is the case.

The governmentality thesis in a nutshell

Governmentality is different from government and from governance. Government is simply the executive power of the (modern) state. It develops policies, programmes and regulations to make sure that the legal framework of a society is maintained and the will of the legislative authority (which in a democracy is usually deemed to be 'the people') is actualized. Governance or administration (which can be treated as synonymous) is the manner in which governments act. In this sense it can be contrasted with commerce, which is the way in which markets operate. Governance entails forms of regulation and control, including interventions by means of non-market based allocations of resources (finance, goods, services, people, information, space, time etc.).

Governmentality, however, is an *ethos* (the term 'mentality' is deliberately used in this respect) of governance. It is one in which the allocation of resources goes beyond a transaction between two parties but entails a 'binding' of the receiver to the provider. Governmentality thus implies a discursive transaction alongside a material one. It entails modes of subjugation, the formation of specific subjects-of-governance (Foucault 1980). The state subsidizes a particular activity, but the subsidized must fulfil certain requirements and make themselves available for continued scrutiny and inspection (surveillance). That is, governmentality exists because governance entails the ability to permit; to provide as well as to prohibit and to withhold. Beyond that, it also incorporates the ability to impose sanctions (punishment). Practically speaking, governmentality depends on the gathering, manufacturing, engineering, processing, storing, retrieving, manipulating and evaluating of large amounts of data (e.g. population statistics, epidemiological data, school exams, police records).

Governmentality, however, is most effective when it entails an 'internalization' of governance by the governed (e.g. subsidized). This internalization is the work of discipline (Foucault 1977).

When applied to risk, governmentality refers to the way in which specific definitions of what constitutes a risk, who constitutes a risk and who is at risk are distributed discursively (see Mairal 2006). To a large extent, governmentality relies on technoscientific expertise. According to Lupton (1999: 87), the specific dimension that risk brings to governmentality is that it gives licence to governmental intervention and regulation. For example, the suspected existence of a risk triggers the gathering, processing and evaluating of data of both populations-of-risk (e.g. the poor, the marginal) as well as populations-at-risk (e.g. the 'vulnerable'). It is for this reason that Lupton (ibid.) refers to risk as a 'moral technology'.

An additional feature of risk is that it implies a calculation. Unlike danger, risk engenders a sense of 'knowing' and thereby calls upon a relationship between information and anticipation (Adam and Van Loon 2000). This is of huge importance when considering governmentality as a moral technology (primarily risk-avoidance). Because risks are predicated upon information, 'to be informed' becomes a moral obligation. The nature of this moral obligation can be externally imposed (e.g. as in law and social norms) but also subjectively internalized (e.g. through associations between risk and blame (Douglas 1992)), and often through a combination of both. Data gathering, processing and evaluation are thus part of a moral-technological enterprise that binds subjectivities to systems of governance.

Students of Foucault have applied the governmentality thesis with particular effectiveness to nineteenth-century Europe[2] where the emergent nation state started to deploy techniques of regulation and control to separate specific 'dangerous groups' and target them with particular modes of governance (e.g. Donzelot 1977; de Regt 1984). The articulation of dangerousness meant that groups could be singled out for specific treatment as a means of securing social order and managing public health. In this sense, the institutionalization of modern society, which took considerable shape in the nineteenth century, closely resembled Foucault's analysis (1977) of incarceration as the prevailing mode of punishment in modern society. Indeed, the system of the 'panopticon' (omnipresent vision) which was used as a means of managing prisons was being effectively exported to hospitals, schools, barracks and factories (Deleuze 1992). With the expanding capacity to gather, process, store and manage data (and the development of statistics and statistical analyses), the panopticon became pervasive throughout society itself. The deployment of risk is a means of identifying specific targets of surveillance and punishment. This has two components: on the one hand it enables a focused allocation of resources to specific social groups as subjects of risk; on the other hand it can serve as a general means to discipline entire populations as subjects at risk. This will be illustrated with regard to teenage sexual risk behaviour in the UK.

Teenage sexual risk behaviour in the UK

It is widely known that the UK has the worst statistics regarding teenage sexual health in Western Europe. It is for this reason that the British government launched its 'Teenage Pregnancy Strategy' (TPS) in 1999. The main aim of the TPS was to halve the teenage conception rates among under-18s by the year 2010.

> The Strategy has four major components: 1) a national media awareness campaign via independent radio and teenage magazines, 2) joined up action to ensure that action is co-ordinated nationally and locally across all relevant statutory and voluntary agencies, 3) better prevention through improving sex and relationships education and improving access to contraception and sexual health services and 4) support for teenage parents to reduce their long term risk of social exclusion by increasing the proportion returning to education, training or employment.
>
> (Teenage Pregnancy Strategy Evaluation (henceforth TPSE) 2005: i)

From this we can deduce that the TPS is based on certain *assumptions*: (a) young people are ignorant about and/or careless with sexual risks; (b) governmental involvement needs more coordination; and (c) existing teenage mothers need help to become more economically independent. Of these, only one (a) can be said to have any immediate relationship with the causes of teenage pregnancy. Simply put, the UK government believes that (female) British teenagers are more likely to become pregnant because they are ill-informed, ignorant and 'careless'. This is not a new assumption and has been central to the UK's sexual health provision for over three decades. The introduction of sex education in the early 1970s can be seen as a prime example of the way in which teenage sexual risk behaviour became an issue of governance. No longer was it deemed to be the responsibility of parents to ensure their children were able to engage in proper sexual relationships. Teenage sexuality had to be governed in a more binding and disciplined way. Ignorance was no longer bliss but became a sin, and young people were given the moral obligation to know (Haywood 1996; Lear 1997; Monk 1998).

It is by no means clear that the introduction of sex education in schools in the UK has had any lasting dampening effect on teenage pregnancy rates. As Figure 4.1 shows, the drop in teenage pregnancies had already started, despite the fact that the legalisation of abortion in 1967 created a few 'peak years' in teenage conceptions (Kane and Wellings 1999; Van Loon 2003). Moreover, the drop could also be explained by a decline in teenage girls entering into marriage. In any case, towards the end of the 1970s, the downward trend in teenage pregnancies ended and the rates started to rise again. Throughout the 1980s there were fluctuations in teenage pregnancy rates; and in the 1990s the rates started to increase slightly year by year.

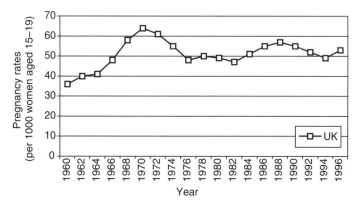

Figure 4.1 Teenage pregnancy rates in the UK 1960–1996 (source: Kane and Wellings 1999: 47)

The AIDS awareness campaigns that emerged in the mid 1980s were based on highlighting the seriousness of sexual risks and promoting 'safe sex'; however, if we look at the statistics we notice that, despite these highly public campaigns, teenagers continued to engage in sexual risk behaviour. The year 1998 marked a peak year in teenage pregnancy rates, which since then have started to recede again slightly. Therefore, when the TPS was activated in 2000, teenage pregnancy rates were already no longer increasing.

The costs of the first five years of the TPS have been estimated at 167.6 million GBP, of which 90 million GBP was direct government contribution (TPSE 2005: 57). The cost of a single teenage conception is estimated as 1,814 GBP per pregnancy. While it is difficult to ascertain how many pregnancies have actually been averted as a consequence of the TPS, it is evident that between 1999 and 2003 there was a moderate decrease of teenage pregnancy rates as measured against 1998, which was a statistical 'peak year' (TPSE 2005: 44). The Teenage Pregnancy Strategy Evaluation estimates that an overall decline of 2.3% means that the costs for averting a pregnancy would be 4,623 GBP, which is still more than twice as high as the costs of a pregnancy.

The fact that the UK government's TPS has not been cost effective and is unlikely to be so in the future, however, has not dampened the spirits of those who advocate it as the best way to reduce teenage sexual risk behaviour and improve teenage sexual health. Indeed, nearly all the recommendations made by the authors of the TPSE point towards a further intensification of the efforts outlined by the TPS, with an expansion of state involvement in and regulation of sexual health provision, abortion and contraception facilitation, sex education and risk-awareness raising campaigns.

It is quite clear then that risk management does not have to make economic sense in order to prevail. This means that we need to look beyond simple notions of outcome-oriented 'effectiveness'. Instead, we need to analyse the way(s) in which the concept of risk can be invoked to develop forms of governmentality and regulation that fail to satisfy a simple economic rationale of cost-effectiveness. It logically follows that policy strategies do not necessarily require a watertight economic basis of risk assessment to be deemed successful. Instead the case of teenage sexual risks reveals that a looser definition of risk is far more conducive to developing forms of governmentality that are ubiquitous and pervasive and conform much more closely to an agenda of social and cultural engineering.

A second focus of this chapter is on the way in which the TPS embraces a highly instrumentalist view of technology which forms the cornerstone of its risk management strategy. This instrumentalism is a central tenet of what Beck (1997) referred to as 'subpolitics'. Whereas the TPS is having only very modest effects (and even these are highly debatable) on reducing teenage pregnancies, its wider embedding in sexual health provision in the UK suggests far greater problems regarding the effectiveness of managing teenage sexual risk behaviour. The argument I am pursuing is that the nature of governmentality regarding teenage sexual risk behaviour entails a transformation of sexual subjectivity that may actually have rendered young people *more vulnerable* to risk.

The evidence for this is more easily found in a second set of indicators of sexual risk behaviour: sexually transmitted infections (STIs). Whereas the TPS can be said to have had no tangible impact on reducing teenage pregnancies, its implementation may have coincided with significant *increase* in incidence of sexual risk behaviour (see Figure 4.2).

The figures in Figure 4.2 are derived from the Genito-Urinary Medicine (GUM) clinics who are involved in the diagnosis and treatment of STIs in the UK. In other words, they only contain data of people *diagnosed* with STIs. If we take a longer historical perspective, in this case focusing on chlamydia which is the most common STI in the UK at the moment, we can discern the pattern shown in Figure 4.3.

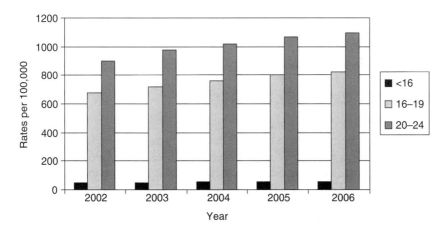

Figure 4.2 STI rates in the UK 2002–2006 (source: Health Protection Agency 2005)

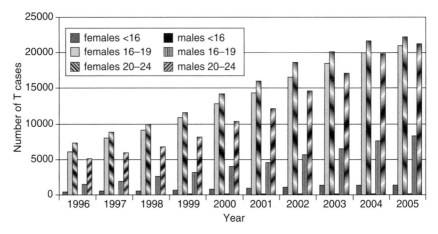

Figure 4.3 Chlamydia in the UK by age and sex (source: Health Protection Agency 2005)

The figures in Figure 4.3 show that the introduction of the TPS in 2000 has not led to a reduction of the incidence of chlamydia amongst young people. All selected cohorts have continued to show an upward tendency. Two contrasting arguments have been deployed to explain these increases: (a) it is evidence of an increased engagement of young people in sexual risk behaviour; (b) it is the consequence of a better screening of STIs amongst young people. These explanations have a direct bearing on how one evaluates the effectiveness of the TPS. If (a) is more accurate it means that young people are engaged in more sexual risk behaviour and that the TPS is thus a clear failure; if (b) is more accurate then it is an indication of its success as more young people are seeking treatment. Indeed, this shows that risk definitions are deeply political and epidemiological data can be used to support two completely contrasting arguments. This, I would argue, is the core of why governmentality requires subpolitics. Visualization of a potential risk is never enough on its own. Its significance has to be determined discursively and its value has to be established both economically and strategically.

Governmentality and vulnerability

It is remarkable that little attention has been paid to the complex life worlds of British teenagers in the formulation of the TPS. Instead, the strategy is heavily biased towards expanding the realm of governance: creating institutions, agencies, discourses, protocols, directives and policy heuristics. Needless to say, the suggested ineffectiveness of the TPS to produce any significant reduction in teenage pregnancy rates and the blatant failure of measures designed to stem the increasing incidence of STIs both highlight the extent to which the products of the TPS may not have affected the 'relevances' that govern young people's experiences.

However, perhaps we should not be looking for the primary effectiveness of TPS in the realm of improving teenage sexual health. Instead, one could argue that the TPS has been highly effective in another way; namely, in creating an expansive apparatus for social engineering. The social engineering takes place at the 'front desk' of sexual health services, for example clinics, leaflets, websites, sex education and media campaigns. However, this social engineering is supported by shifts in discursive articulations of governance itself. This has primarily taken place in the 'back offices' in the form of shifting alliances between health care and educational apparatuses. The allocation of resources to such forms of 'coordination' and 'joined up action' entails the continuous calibration of the three major forces that enable the anchoring of 'risk' in social institutions: visualization by 'technoscience' (e.g. sexual health expertise), signification by media, educational and political apparatuses and valorization by commercial, para-commercial (state-funded or subsidized) as well as legal means.[3] The Teenage Pregnancy Strategy can thus be seen as an example of the way in which governmentality operates through particular risks as a continuous process. It builds upon already existing infrastructures of health communication and sex education, for instance, whilst expanding the institutional infrastructure for the delivery of both policy programmes and information to the general population and teenagers in particular (Monk 1998).

One crucial way in which governmentality operates is by creating specific categories it can deploy to manage, regulate and control populations. What matters here is the ability to identify 'subjects-at-risk' and 'subjects-of-risk'. The first category is often the population at large; the second category is a distinctive target group which have some causal responsibility for the endangerment of the former (Lupton 1999: 114; Mairal 2006). In the case of sexual risk behaviour, certain groups of young people have been singled out as 'subjects of risk'; these are primarily young women whose social situation or level of awareness makes them most vulnerable to engagement in sexual risk behaviour (Lear 1997).

Vulnerability is a specific label that can be deployed to justify targeted actions towards/against specific groups of people. It enables governmentality to adopt the cloak of 'concern and care' or what Foucault (1982) termed 'pastoral power'. Targeted regulation and control are required because these vulnerable people need to be protected against the risks and, quite often, against themselves. Such a view suggests that vulnerable people suffer because they fail to constitute themselves as responsible citizens; the realization of their subjectivity is marred either by personal deficiencies (e.g. ignorance) or structural impositions (e.g. social exclusion, sexism). As with interpreting epidemiological data, the emphasis on either personal or structural deficiencies is a matter of politics. This again highlights that governmentality is not a purely 'neutral' process driven by the need for effectiveness and efficiency, but retains a sense of agency in the form of differences in intentionality, ethical preferences and prejudices.

What is needed, therefore, is a more thorough contextual analysis of the social and political environment in which the governmentality of teenage sexual risk behaviour emerged. The purpose of this is to show that the governmentality perspective on vulnerability and health risks *requires* an analysis of the subpolitical involvement of different sets of actors: experts, lobby groups, politicians, but also those involved in commerce and marketing need to be considered.

Signification and subpolitics

The expert engagement with matters of sexual health might be analysed as an example of the 'subpolitics' of a risk society (Beck 1997). As with so many elements of Beck's expansive conceptual framework (cf. Van Loon 2002a), his concept of subpolitics contains a paradox. On the one hand, Beck deploys it to denote forms of political mobilization 'from below' (that is, from 'civil society', activist groups etc.); on the other hand, Beck (1997: 94–109) refers to an 'undercurrent' of systemic power that operates outside the realms of public scrutiny and accountability. He subsequently poses a distinction between 'simple' (or rule-directed) and 'reflexive' (rule-altering) subpolitics to show how the development of (reflexive) modernity might contain within it a moment of bifurcation when it comes across the point of no return when it either follows the simple route and entrenches itself in institutionalized authoritarianism, or it follows the reflexive route of innovation and democratic revitalization.

Sexual health expertise is indeed subpolitical in both senses. On the one hand, it embraces the institutional mantra of science, invoking the factual and disinterested language of clinical expertise; on the other hand it embraces an ethos of sexual reformism. Under the first heading, it has effectively established itself as a key component of public sexual health provision both in the realm of clinical as well as educational practices. Under the second heading, it promotes a distinctive normative vision of sexual health. In the Western world, sexual reformism is indeed a social movement and closely affiliated with, for example, the Birth Control League, Planned Parenthood Foundation, Mary Stopes International or the UK-based Brook Advisory Centres.

The point is simply that the subpolitical status of sexual health expertise enables a translation of what in essence were once *ideological* articulations into *disciplinary* ones. For example, issues regarding 'good sexual practices' are articulated in terms of the disciplinary dispositions of thoughtfulness and risk-aversion and contrasted with the ideological 'sex-negative culture'. Indeed, the Brook Advisory Clinics website, whose mission is to offer 'free and confidential sexual health advice and contraception to young people up to the age of 25' (http://www.brook.org.uk/content/M1_gotobrook.asp), advises young people when they are not sure about having sex in the following way:

> If you're unsure about having sex, it might be worth talking to a counsellor about your feelings. Remember that there are different ways of giving each other pleasure, apart from full sex. It's important not to feel pressurised into doing anything that you're not ready for. If you are thinking of having sex,

then it's also important to get advice about contraception to avoid pregnancy and sexually transmitted infections.

(http://www.brook.org.uk/content/M3_4_sexandrelationships.asp)

Again we can see how specific opinions about 'good' or 'normal' sexuality (which are tied in with the liberal view of a self-sufficient self-knowing individual) are embedded in a language of expertise. The hyperlinks guide the reader further back into the 'service provision packages' that the Brook offers to its clients, generating a self-referential discursive formation that effectively replaces more critical and rule-altering forms of reflexivity. The question 'what do I do?' is not really answered in a substantive manner. Instead, the hypothetical teenager looking for advice is told that s/he has to make up his/her own mind and decide when s/he is ready for sex (Tincknell *et al.* 2003). However, the normative indifference regarding 'readiness for sex' does not stretch to issues of risk and safety. Indeed, here the advice is an unequivocal endorsement of risk aversion via contraception and institutional surveillance. It perfectly fits Beck and Beck-Gernsheim's (2002) individualization thesis in which they suggest that a main consequence of the emergence of risk has been that institutions have been able to successfully divert the onus of accountability onto the individual (also see Wilkinson 2001: 30).

When turning to the Birth Control League's dual concerns over the nature of social deprivation and women's oppression, we can see a similar translation of ideological concerns into disciplinary ones. In identifying high birth rates as the cause of both poverty and women's oppression, Margaret Sanger occupies an ideological position with regard to the nature of adequate moral conduct in sexual reproduction. That is to say, the normativity of her discourse is politically motivated. However, when the contraceptive pill was made available for general public use in the early 1960s, this normativity shifted to a more instrumentalist position as expressed in the perceived need for women to be educated about how it should be used. This is a technological normativity that relates to the function of contraception as an instrument of birth control and not on the rights and wrongs of uses and consequences of artificial birth control itself.

The task of providing technological or instrumental normativity was quickly assumed by 'sexual health experts'. Whereas this process of knowledge transfer may have entailed some expansion of women's general understanding of fertility and the reproductive cycle (although it could be argued, such knowledge has to be far more extensive in so-called 'natural' family planning methods), the focus on the contraceptive pill meant that this knowledge-transfer mainly involved the generation of an awareness that women's reproduction can now be regulated as a matter of habit rather than deliberate intervention, and can thus become part of the rhythms of everyday life.

An important aspect of the provision of the contraceptive pill is that it is only made available upon doctor's prescription and thus requires women to visit their GPs and engage in consultations over their sexual and reproductive health. Such consultations often involve both verbal and practical 'check ups' which render women's bodies further visible to the medical gaze. As always, such medicalization is presented under the banner of 'care', hence invoking the pastoral power of paternalistic governmentality for 'one's own good' (e.g. Martin 1987).

With the introduction of the contraceptive pill, the intrusion of the medical gaze into everyday lives, especially of women, rapidly expanded. As the advantages of the pill were extended to that of regulating the entire sexual hormonal balance of women, it was also increasingly prescribed as part of the treatment of other 'dysfunctionalities' such as premenstrual syndrome (PMS) and irregular menstrual cycles (Martin 1987). Such 'discoveries' of additional benefits of the pill were generally greeted with enthusiasm by the mass media, perhaps because it vindicated the popular perception that regulating sexuality by means of medico-technological interventions was a good (perhaps even natural) thing. It was only when the first signals of negative side effects came to light that such general endorsements of the contraceptive pill were balanced with more critical questioning.

Foucault's (1963) concept of medicalization (also see Lupton 1994 and Martin 1987) shows how the medical gaze provided a crucial vehicle for the expansion of administration onto as well as into the body. Through the systematic application of medical technoscience, bodies could be rendered 'transparent' and thereby manipulated for the maximization of 'functionality' and discipline. Such docile, useful bodies were not only productive in an economic sense, but also enabled an expansion of social ordering that was conducive to an extension of rationalization to the minute details of everyday life.

Public health is clearly a main domain in which the personal becomes political, but not in the sense advocated by feminists (Hanisch 1970; Morgan 1970). In contrast, medicalization hardly involved any agency or subjective autonomy (also see Lupton 1999). It is a highly systemic and abstract apparatus containing an extensive repertoire of statistical techniques and discursive practices in which specific subjectivities (in the form of categories) are produced with a high degree of regularity and control. Medicalization has been essential in the establishment of the individual as an administrative unit of the political organization of civil society (Beck 1992; Lupton 1999).

Governmentality and commodification

The third dimension of governmentality is the process of valorization which, in capitalist societies, is primarily accomplished via the market; that is, value is generated by its attachment to commodity forms. The concerns over overpopulation, reproductive health and women's emancipation may be in essence ideologically motivated; however, in contemporary Western societies the issues they refer to are no longer perceived as 'matters of opinion' but simply accepted as 'matters of fact'. The successful transfer of sexuality from the realm of politics to that of sub-politics, however, could not have taken place without a substantive infusion of material resources. It is in this respect that the Foucauldian doctrine of disciplinary power is perhaps less adequate as it tends to dismiss 'economic motivation' (let alone the issue of economic interest).

Beck's risk society thesis (1992) is also rather brief on the economics of risk, although this is not necessarily excluded from its framework. One of the crucial dimensions of risk has *from the start* been the ability to *capitalize* on anxieties and fears. This was already the case in the pre-modern era (Bernstein 1996), but when it became dislodged from a religious worldview, our understanding of risk also shifted from fate to chance and the mood changed from general resignation to a bifurcation of anxiety and opportunism to the extent that we now seem to live in a culture in which both extreme cases of risk avoidance and risk-entrepreneurialism can exist side-by-side (Lupton 1999; Wilkinson 2001).

As already stipulated, when discussing the UK's TPS, teenage sexual health is big business. To be able to spend 167.6 million GBP in four years has massive consequences in terms of employment but also investments in specific commodities. Hence, when concerns over specific risks are voiced (e.g. by the eugenics movements in the 1920s and 1930s, or by sexual health clinics today), these are almost immediately translated into appeals for increased resourcing for 'health expertise provision' in the form of 'family planning services' such as contraception and abortion.[4] It is for this reason that the shift from ideology to governmentality is essential. Whereas ideology (sexual reformism) is always partisan, partial and perspectival, governmentality (e.g. through sexual health expertise) can always assume the voice of reason, objectivity and neutrality because it represents a 'view from nowhere'.

It would therefore be misleading to suggest that these developments in sexual health expertise simply emerged out of either the emancipatory zeal of modernity or the more cynical and instrumental motives of the nation state and industrial capital. This is because, like all technoscience, sexual health expertise requires a constant stream of resources to be able to develop and maintain itself. The resourcing of technoscience is unfortunately one of the most underestimated aspects within both science and technology studies as well as risk studies. It is, however, an essential condition of its existence and, as a result, we should expect that a considerable portion of the available energy within sexual health expertise is being devoted to generating the necessary resources for its survival.

Ideology-becoming-expertise then is never merely an epiphenomenon of power or domination; it is also a pivotal part of strategies of resource allocation. Hence, what comes under the banner of 'health education' is not simply an arsenal of techniques made available to the general public to enhance their health and quality of life, it is also a means by which people's dependence on technoscience is affirmed and/or strengthened. The education provision of sexual health teaches people that they should apply birth control technologies and how to use them. These technologies are associated with commodities and products that have to be bought, and are being manufactured and sold at a profit; even if insurance companies (who also make a profit) and state-governed schemes (funded by taxation) seem to be paying for it. Sexual health education has also succeeded in redirecting a massive shift of resources towards the marketing of 'sexual' commodities (knowledge, information and contraceptives as well as pleasure-enhancement devices) which themselves generate huge profits for the pharmaceutical and para-pharmaceutical industries as well as the 'sexual pleasure' industries (related to the 'expert' knowledge of 'how to please' which is associated with the sexual reform ideology).

Pharmaceutical companies' involvement in the development of the contraceptive pill, manufacturers of condoms, but also professional expertise and service industries such as Mary Stopes abortion clinics and Brooks Advisory Centres, has often been neglected in reflections on the sexual revolution. Indeed the sexual health services industry has greatly benefited financially from 'the sexual revolution' in the sense that this entailed the expansion of their markets and potential clientele. It is remarkable that, in public debates over sexual health expertise, this financial dimension is generally ignored in favour of their alleged contributions to the common good. This, in turn, enables such organizations to present their work as if it is for the public benefit and as if they are neutral and objective agents in public debates over sexual ideologies.[5]

The subpolitical reconstruction of the so-called sexual revolution has successfully appropriated the commercial infrastructure of sexual health expertise and turned its cold hard economic rationale into a (moral) technology of care. By drawing resources mainly from the public sector, there is no immediate visibility of commercial interests, yet someone needs to be paid to develop curricular material, in the same way that 'free condoms' have to be bought from condom manufacturers and contraceptive pills from pharmaceutical companies.

In fact, one could argue that the commodification of sexuality has been the major factor in a process that has been recently dubbed as the 'sexualisation of society' (UNICEF 2001). This process is marked by a subtle form of alienation. Young people are at once active participants in this sexualization and at the same time at risk from it. Their vulnerability is exploited both in economic terms, through the marketing and commodification of sexual subjectivities, as well as in governmental terms through their being rendered 'transparent' by invasive technologies of surveillance, discipline and control. It is as if young people are unwittingly participating in their own risk behaviour, because at once they are being seen as hormone-crazed, unstoppable, curious consumers of sex; yet at the same time they are portrayed as ill-informed, ignorant, misled by religious and conservative traditions and victims of 'mixed messages'. The messages sent to them as part of the TPS are supposed to terminate this alienation and produce informed, responsible, sexual citizens who can decide for themselves what it is they want in terms of sex.

However, by placing so much emphasis on information provision and access to facilities, the vulnerability of young people is actually reproduced rather than diminished. Young people are affirmed in their incompleteness and their alienation because the modes of 'responsible sexual subjectivity' are discursively engineered by a combination of expertise, governmentality and commodification. The entire TPS is devoid of a phenomenological grounding in what it means to be a teenager in a sexualized society. In its media campaigns targeting teenagers, such as the website www.rethinking.co.uk, it merely uses an apparent 'mimesis' of coolness, deploying 'direct teen speak' and modes of enunciation that emphasize pseudo-equality (see Tincknell *et al.* 2003), whilst failing to ask the basic question: are teenagers engaged in sexual risk behaviour because they are ignorant?

At the same time, voices speaking against the TPS are marginalized sometimes by means of ridicule, more often simply by a wall of silence. Hence, it is possible that nearly 170 million pounds can be spent without apparent success, yet so little time spent on the fundamental question whether this is money well spent. This is inherent in a technological culture in which expertise, governmentality and commodification are integrated into a seemingly perfect symbiosis (all singing from the same hymn sheet that 'there is no alternative').[6] Such a symbiosis tolerates no dissent and ruthlessly subjugates all differences to its own strongly policed version of 'diversity'.

Conclusion

From the perspective of governmentality, we can see how 'health risks' can be reconfigured as a specific realm of subpolitical intervention. Public health often entails issues which seem to go beyond party-political divides. How could anyone be against the health of a nation or the world for that matter? Hence, health risks provide excellent opportunities to transform partisan politics into generic politics and, beyond that, into matters of national and even global concern. In enabling a subpolitical reconfiguration of health risks, vulnerability is a crucial modality. The attachment of vulnerability to a section of the population renders them available for surveillance and care (a form of pastoral power, often seen as benevolent). At the same time, this 'rendering available' availing can be understood as a form of disciplinary power; it entails a specific formation of subjectivity. The subject of health risks is a vulnerable subject in both senses; it is a subject whose integrity is compromised and whose claim to autonomy is questioned.

The strength of the governmentality thesis has been tested by the specific case study of teenage sexual risk behaviour. Teenagers have been widely conceptualized as a vulnerable social group. This is especially the case in relation to sexual health issues. In the UK, teenage sexual risk behaviour has been a primary concern of the Labour government since it came to power in 1997, resulting in the 'Teenage Pregnancy Strategy' (TPS). Since its introduction, the UK teenage pregnancy rate has only marginally decreased. The TPS has not created a significant shift in the fluctuating trends of teenage pregnancy rates. Moreover, its implementation has coincided with a continued rise in STI rates amongst young people.

A reasonable question any policy evaluation might ask is whether it is worthwhile continuing the TPS given its huge expenses thus far and lack of tangible success. One may be hugely surprised to find that such a debate has not taken place yet, at least not in public. Despite a clear lack of any convincing evidence that the TPS is actually having any significant effect in reducing teenage pregnancies, there is little indication that the TPS will be revised, or even that there is any discussion of an alternative strategy. Indeed, the absence of a discussion itself suggests the strong presence of a subpolitical momentum. What we are dealing with here is not a simple, synoptic rational political process in which an intervention is subjected to a cost–benefit analysis to decide whether it should continue. What we have instead is clear evidence of the strength of Ulrich Beck's (1992) risk society thesis. It testifies to the pervasiveness of risk as a means to distribute resources and entitlements. It is by continuing to stress the vulnerability of young people, through for example epidemiological data, that further support for the TPS is being mobilized. The data do not reveal the failure of TPS, but are being called upon to support its necessity. This is because, in the risk society, risks set to work a rather different type of economics.

Especially in the realm of health care, it is the way in which certain risks can be deployed to mobilize public concern that determines their effectiveness in attracting material, symbolic as well as political resources. As AIDS activists know all too well, when HIV/AIDS was primarily understood to be a gay-related illness, it hardly stirred public concern; but when it became redefined as a generic STI, which also had the potential to affect heterosexuals, it turned into a huge worldwide public health concern as well as a highly lucrative domain of pharmaceutical R&D, not to mention an opportunity-rich field for developing expertise and awareness-raising activism. Most significant for the issue of teenage sexual risk behaviour, however, is the way in which HIV/AIDS enabled a radical intervention into subjectivity. It inaugurated a new subject, a universally vulnerable subject, a subject-at-risk and a subject-of-risk; this subject is the sexual citizen of a society where sexual practices have to be 'well informed' and 'scrutinized'. Sexual citizenship will 'have to' be taught in schools, because it does not come naturally, or even through existing modes of socialization.

It is at this critical intersection that health risks and vulnerabilities operate within complex discursive settings. There is no need to deny or even question the existence of risks, as the actuality of risk is never distinct from its virtuality. Something is a risk, solely by virtue of it being perceivable as such; the durability of a risk perception is directly linked to its stabilization within networks of articulations (Van Loon 2002a). Although science often provides a powerful set of articulations which can strengthen or undermine the durability of a risk, it does not have a monopoly of risk-definition.[7] In other words, whereas the allocation of risk-subjects, that is as subjects of risk or subjects at risk, is ultimately a deeply political issue, the ability to maintain lasting risk-perceptions and risk-definitions rests on a range of other factors, many of which may not appear to be political at all.

Perhaps future research in this area needs to engage more directly with the counterfactual hypothesis that what we are dealing with is not governmentality at all, but rather 'ideology'. That is to say, the British government's attachment to the TPS is perhaps not so much to do with surveillance and discipline, but with social reproduction within the confines of contemporary global capitalism. Indeed, one could argue that the deployment of TPS is a means to facilitate the further commodification of sex, which has also been dubbed 'the sexualisation of society' (e.g.

UNICEF 2001). Indeed, the latter perspective comes close to what Lodziak (1995), using Marcuse and Gortz, has referred to as 'a manipulation of needs'.

It could be argued that these contrasting perspectives, that is, governmentality and neo-Marxism, might both have something critical to offer to understanding teenage sexual risk behaviour as an area of governance. Whilst the first exposes the hidden dimensions of regulation and control as a formation of distinctive, docile subjectivities, the latter reveals that beneath the veil of 'pastoral power' there are cold, hard economic interests that often need ideological make-up to appear acceptable and legitimate. Albeit from different angles, both perspectives point towards a convergence between governmentality and commodification, marking what might be a rather decisive turning within the risk society towards a highly invasive form of social engineering. This engineering takes place through articulating and distributing distinctive vulnerabilities – both in terms of individual bodies and populations (biopower) – although remaining fully compatible with the logic of capitalism.

Notes

1 Although Foucault himself did not write about risks as such, his historical and theoretical analyses of psychiatry, medicine, prisons, sexuality etc. all have clear relevance to risk research, as he was dealing with the way in which 'anomalies' (madness, illness, crime, homosexuality) were being managed within modern society.
2 However, see Susan Craddock's (2000) excellent analysis of similar principles applied to the management of tuberculosis in San Francisco for a non-European example.
3 See Van Loon (2002b) for a more detailed discussion of these three functions.
4 Whereas it is no coincidence that the majority of recent initiatives by UNESCO have focused on 'family planning and sexual health' of so-called 'Third World' countries, it is rather remarkable that such clearly racially biased policy initiatives are not scrutinized more critically by (anti-racist) political activists on the Left.
5 It is for this reason that such organizations are allowed to be omnipresent in government-sponsored information provision about sexual health. For example, on the TPS website, direct links to the following organizations are present on the home page: the Brook, Family Planning Association, Marie Stopes and the British Pregnancy Advisory Service. Whereas they all have strong ideational motivations regarding sexual reform, linked to various forms of civic activism, none of these are seen to be overtly 'political'. This is because they are all strongly subpolitical, embracing the mantra of neutral scientific expertise, pastoral power and institutionalized discipline.
6 The symbiosis between capitalism, governmentality and the subpolitics of the progressive social forces of the women's movements, gay and lesbian movements and civil rights movements was quite opportunistic. Suddenly it seemed as if capitalism and modernity were – by their very nature – on the side of human emancipation; and this provided such a powerful – albeit rather volatile – alliance that it was almost self-evident that promoting a commodified sexuality was inherently good. This also explains the close alliance between so-called 'hippie culture', experimental performance art and the rising porn industry.
7 Leaving aside the question whether it ever had such a monopoly, the loss of a commanding presence of science in relations of risk-definition (Beck 2000) is a key feature of the risk society (Adam and Van Loon 2000).

References

Adam, B. and Van Loon, J. (2000) 'Introduction', in B. Adam, U. Beck and J. Van Loon (eds) *The Risk Society and Beyond: Critical Issues for Social Theory*, pp. 1–31. London: Sage.

Beck, U. (1992) *Risk Society: Towards a New Modernity.* Trans. M. Ritter. London: Sage.

Beck, U. (1997) *The Reinvention of Politics: Rethinking Modernity in the Global Social Order.* Cambridge: Polity.

Beck, U. (2000) 'Risk society revisited: Theory, politics and research programmes', in B. Adam, U. Beck and J. Van Loon (eds) *The Risk Society and Beyond: Critical Issues for Social Theory.* London: Sage, pp. 211–29.

Beck, U. and Beck-Gernsheim, E. (2002) *Individualization: Institutionalized Individualism and its Social and Political Consequences.* London: Sage.

Bernstein, P. (1996) *Against the Gods: The Remarkable Story of Risk.* New York: John Wiley.

Burchell, G., Gordon, C. and Miller, P. (eds) (1991) *The Foucault Effect: Studies in Governmentality.* Hemel Hempstead: Harvester Wheatsheaf.

Craddock, S. (2000) *City of Plagues: Disease, Poverty and Deviance in San Francisco.* Minneapolis: University of Minnesota Press.

Deleuze, G. (1992) 'Postscript on the societies of control', *October* 59: 3–7.

de Regt, A. (1984) *Arbeidersgezinnen en Beschavingsarbeid: Ontwikkelingen in Nederland 1870–1940.* Amsterdam: Boom Meppel.

Donzelot, J. (1977) *La Police des Familles.* Paris: Édition de Minuit.

Douglas, M. (1992) *Risk and Blame: Essays in Cultural Theory.* London: Routledge.

Foucault, M. (1963) *Naissance de la clinique: Une archéologie du regard médical.* Paris: Presses Universitaires de France.

Foucault, M. (1977) *Discipline and Punish: The Birth of the Prison.* New York: Vintage.

Foucault, M. (1979) *The History of Sexuality: An Introduction* (Volume 1). New York: Vintage.

Foucault, M. (1980) *Power/Knowledge: Selected Interviews and Other Writings 1972–1977.* New York: Pantheon Books.

Foucault, M. (1982) 'Subject and power: Afterword', in H.L. Dreyfus and P. Rabinow (eds) *Michel Foucault: Beyond Structuralism and Hermeneutics.* Chicago: University of Chicago Press.

Hanisch, C. (1970) 'The personal is political', *Notes from the Second Year. Women's Liberation: Major Writings of the Radical Feminists.* New York: Radical Feminism, pp. 204–5.

Haywood, C. (1996) 'Sex education policy and the regulation of young people's sexual practice', *Educational Review* 48(2): 121–9.

Health Protection Agency (2005) 'Epidemiological data – HIV and sexually transmitted infections'. Available at http://www.hpa.org.uk/infections/topics_az/hiv_and_sti/epidemiology/epidemiology.htm (accessed January 2006).

Kane, R. and Wellings, K. (1999) *Reducing the Rate of Teenage Conceptions. An International Review of the Evidence: Data from Europe.* London: Health Education Authority.

Lear, D. (1997) *Sex and Sexuality: Risk and Relationships in the Age of AIDS.* London: Sage.

Lodziak, C. (1995) *Manipulating Needs: Capitalism and Culture.* London: Pluto.

Lupton, D. (1994) *Medicine as Culture: Illness, Disease and the Body in Western Societies.* London: Sage.

Lupton, D. (1999) *Risk.* London: Routledge.

Mairal, G. (2006) 'Narratives of risk'. Paper presented at *Riskcom 2006.* Göteborg, 30 August–2 September.

Martin, E. (1987) *The Woman in the Body: A Cultural Analysis of Reproduction.* Milton Keynes: Open University Press.

Monk, D. (1998) 'Sex education and the problematisation of teenage pregnancy: A genealogy of law and governance', *Social and Legal Studies: An International Journal* 7: 239–60.

Morgan, R. (ed.) (1970) *Sisterhood is Powerful: An Anthology of Writings from the Women's Liberation Movement.* New York: Vintage.

Nicoll, A., Catchpole, M., Cliffe, S., Hughes, G., Simms, I. and Thomas, D. (1999) 'Sexual health of teenagers in England and Wales: Analysis of national data', *British Medical Journal* 318 (15 May): 1321–2.

Teenage Pregnancy Strategy Evaluation Research Team (2005) *TPSE Teenage Pregnancy Strategy Evaluation: Final Report Synthesis.* London: Department of Health.

Tincknell, E., Chambers, D. and Van Loon, J. (2003) 'Begging for it: "New femininities", social agency and moral discourse in contemporary teenage and men's magazines', *Feminist Media Studies* 3(1): 44–63.

UNICEF (2001) *A League Table of Teenage Births in Rich Nations.* Florence: UNICEF Innocenti Research Centre.

Van Loon, J. (2002a) *Risk and Technological Culture: Towards a Sociology of Virulence.* London: Routledge.

Van Loon, J. (2002b) 'A contagious living fluid: Objectification and assemblage in the history of virology', *Theory, Culture & Society* 19(5/6): 107–24.

Van Loon, J. (2003) *Deconstructing the Dutch Utopia: Sex Education and Teenage Pregnancy in the Netherlands.* London: Family Education Trust.

Wilkinson, I. (2001) *Anxiety in a Risk Society.* London: Routledge.

Chapter 5

Restructuring health care

Developing systems to identify risk and prevent harm

Andy Alaszewski and Kirstie Coxon

In this chapter we examine the ways in which the government in the UK is developing systems within the health service to identify clinical errors and near misses. We note that the government's main response to its increased concern with risk and maintaining public confidence in services has been to increase central regulation using hierarchical authority to ensure professional compliance. However, at the same time the government has sought to develop a system of organisational learning based on front-line staff's willingness to identify and report near misses and clinical errors. In the main part of this chapter, we will use a small empirical case study to explore the ways in which the non-hierarchical reporting system interacts with the dominant hierarchical culture of the British health care system.

Crisis in governance

Risk and uncertainty have become prominent issues and concerns in late modern society. The increasing importance of risk and uncertainty is evident both in the mass media coverage and in more specialised expert discourse. For example, Lupton found that in the *Sydney Morning Herald* in 1992 'risk' was used 2356 times in news stories and 89 times in headlines and by 1997 this had increased to 3488 times in news stories and 118 in headlines (1999: 10). While Heyman in a quantitative analysis of cited mental health literature between 1993 and 2004 found a progressive increase in reference to risk especially in the literature relating to Forensic Mental Disorder (2004: 298).

Sociologists such as Beck (1992) and Giddens (1991) see the development of risk issues as a product of major socio-economic changes within late modern society and focus particularly on the ways in which these changes have increased individual vulnerability. Building on classic sociological analysis of social change, they emphasise the ways in which globalisation has undermined individuals' security. Events in remote and distant parts of the globe can have devastating impacts on local communities. For instance a financial crisis in General Motors in the USA can lead to the closure of a major factory and unemployment in Ellesmere Port, England. At the same time linked changes in the ways in which individuals manage themselves and their personal relations also increase personal insecurity.

Within late modern society individuals cannot rely on traditional and localised mechanisms of trust such as kinship, community and religion for protection but must develop their own personal systems. For example Giddens notes the ways in which individuals create personal networks of friends and develop relationships of intimacy to provide personal security (Giddens 1991: 102). Since modern risks are increasingly generated by human action (e.g. pollution) and their effects no longer restricted to the poor and vulnerable, even the rich and wealthy cannot protect themselves (Beck 1992: 23), so the fear and anxiety they engender permeates the whole of society:

> [Risk] has come to stand as one of the focal points of feelings of fear, anxiety and uncertainty...Massumi argues that individuals in late modernity experience a constant low-level fear, which is vague, not as sharp as panic or localized as hysteria but rather 'A kind of background radiation saturating experience'.
>
> (Lupton 1999: 12)

As Burgess (2006) has pointed out this approach treats risk as an objective threat to individuals and social groups. Less attention is given to the ways in which risk is socially constructed and the ways in which individuals and groups use risk as a resource to achieve specific aims and objectives. Rothstein (2006) argues that concerns about risk do not primarily arise from increased individual vulnerability and anxiety from increasing societal risks but from institutional pressures, especially from regulatory bodies that have a mandate to protect society from particular hazards. If these regulatory bodies fail to identify and prevent disasters they experience major repercussions and are therefore faced with 'institutional risks' such as legal liabilities, personal sanctions and loss of reputation. He argues that

> the contemporary preoccupation with risk stems not from living in a world that is out of control, but rather, paradoxically stems from our attempts to improve our control of the world through a process that myself and my colleague...have termed *risk colonisation.*
>
> (Rothstein 2006: 216)

The development of a regulatory state in the UK can be seen as loss of confidence in systems of governments and methods of managing risk developed in the nineteenth century, especially self-regulation by expert elites such as the professions and city institutions (Moran 2003: 1–11). As Moran notes, the regulatory state is also a risk state, one based on strong private and public sector governance structures to protect citizens from societal risk (Moran 2003: 26–31). Paradoxically these strong structures increase institutional risk as 'failures have to be recorded, potential failures have to be anticipated, and new categories of failure are defined' (Rothstein 2006: 216). To reduce expectations and provide some defence against failure those responsible for governance and regulation engage in 'risk colonisation'; they create technologies to identify and manage risk while stressing the intrinsic limitations of risk management because of the uncertainties inherent in decision making in the real world. As Rothstein notes 'reframing regulatory objects in terms of risk has proved attractive for rationalising the practical limits of what regulation can achieve' (2006: 216).

While the expansion of regulatory agencies within the regulatory state contributes to the reframing of management processes such as decision making in terms of risk, organisations involved in the production of goods and services contribute to this development. Not only are these organisations subject to increased external inspection, audit and control but they are also expected to improve their own self-regulation through enhanced organisational governance. These new systems are designed to create 'zero tolerance', that is to prevent any failure that could harm a service user or member of the public. Some of these incidents would in the past have been seen as unpreventable random events or accidents (Green 1997). Regulation 'is the response to the now instinctive reaction that "something should be done about it"' (Moran 2003: 26). The attempt to prevent such incidents especially when they cannot be concealed means that policy issues become reframed as risk problems. Human services such as health and welfare services traditionally framed decision making and management in terms of meeting client needs but Kemshall notes: 'Risk, particularly an individualized and responsibilized risk, is replacing need as the core principle of social policy formation and welfare delivery' (2002: 1). Kemshall argues that the development of more responsive public services which are 'safety oriented' is reshaping public services. A more responsive public service is not only more exposed to risk as it is expected to reach higher standards often on lower resources, but is also subject to greater scrutiny through audit systems which are often linked to naming and shaming mechanisms.

The development of the regulatory state is reflected both in the development of regulatory agencies and in the restructuring of agencies. The large organisations that developed at the end of the nineteenth century in both the private and public sector mostly used hierarchical structures and bureaucratic processes to control and manage key processes such as decision making. The systems operate effectively in relatively stable conditions in which there is limited innovation and competition and relatively little uncertainty, for example the Ford motor company in the early twentieth century or the National Health Service in the 1950s and 1960s. Increased instability, whether created by market saturation and associated competition as in the case of car production or by government moving from a system of stable administration of policy to a system based on continual policy innovation (Moran 2003), has driven the development of local decentralised systems of management that can respond to changing policies and targets. Paradoxically, changing policies and targets mean that more local units will fail, for example NHS Trusts with no star ratings or schools in special measures. The decentralised system insulates the central executive from failure or disaster in one unit, ensuring blame remains localised and the local managers are sacked and replaced with a new team.

Restructuring governance
in the health care system

The development of the regulatory state is heavily influenced by the emergence of an inquiry culture in which accidents are increasingly classified as man-made disasters (see Turner and Pidgeon 1997) resulting in a cycle of disaster, inquiry and new safety measures, especially increased regulation. This pattern is particularly evident in health and welfare services with the first major 'modern' disasters that occurred in the late 1960s and early 1970s. These initial disasters mainly concerned the failure of the health and social care agencies and the staff they employed to protect vulnerable individuals, for example children, from being harmed by those who should have been protecting them. Initially these failures were not primarily seen in terms of risk management but in terms of organisational or managerial failures. An overview of child protection inquiry reports argued that

> The reports demonstrate that problems can arise where there is lack of clarity about the different contributions of the various agencies and individuals involved...there are problems of overlap where particular functions are held in common by more than one agency...when many people have duties in relation to one family, for responsibility to become blurred and decisions avoided and for vital information to be lost sight of or overlooked.
>
> (DHSS 1982: 5, 17)

In the 1990s inquiry teams increasingly framed failures in terms of risk. The reports identified failures by agencies to protect the public, staff and patients by failing to effectively assess and manage the risks posed. The agencies failed to identify the potential danger of mentally ill service users such as Christopher Clunis, who killed Jonathan Zito on an underground station, and health professionals, for example Beverley Allitt, Harold Shipman and the surgeons at Bristol Royal Infirmary, who harmed the very people they had a duty to protect.

Since recent inquiries have framed issues in terms of risk, their recommendations tend to focus on ways of improving the identification and management of risk. This is evident in 'iconic' inquiries, which have had a major media and policy impact such as the Clunis and the Bristol Inquiries. The Inquiry into care and treatment of Christopher Clunis identified repeated failure of services to uncover the 'real' dangerousness of Clunis as manifest, for example, in his interest in knives and a failure to share information on and take seriously evidence of his violent behaviour. The Inquiry recommended that risk assessment should be improved and that all violent mental health patients should have 'an assessment...as to whether the patient's propensity for violence presents any risk to his own health or safety or to the protection of the public' (*Report of the Inquiry*, 1994, para. 45.1.2).

The disasters in the late 1960s and early 1970s affected mainly vulnerable individuals being cared for in low-tech sectors of health and social care services. The disasters in the 1980s and 1990s increasingly affected patients being treated in the high-tech environment of the district general hospitals. For example there were disasters in cervical screening, breast screening, histopathological diagnosis and gynaecology (Lugon and Secker-Walker 1999: 1). The defining disaster in this series took place at Bristol Royal Infirmary. This disaster was not only horrific – the Inquiry estimated that at least 35 babies died as the result of the incompetence of the cardiac surgeons – but it also indicated the failure of the NHS to respond to a clearly identified risk. Professionals in the hospitals were well aware of the harm being caused; nurses referred to the operating theatre as 'the killing fields' and an anaesthetist tried to 'blow the whistle', alerting senior management in the Trust and wider NHS to the harm being caused. Despite this, operations continued and parents were unaware of the unacceptable risks to which they were exposing their children.

The disaster at Bristol Royal Infirmary can be seen as a watershed. The editor of the *British Medical Journal* (BMJ), writing on the consequences of the disaster in Bristol, entitled his commentary 'All changed, changed utterly' (Smith 1998). The final report of the Bristol Inquiry identified a culture of dangerousness at the hospital which persisted despite whistle blowing:

> The story of the paediatric cardiac surgical service in Bristol is...an account of people who cared greatly about human suffering, and were dedicated and well-motivated. Sadly, some lacked insight and their behaviour was flawed. Many failed to communicate with each other, and to work together effectively for the interests of their patients. There was a lack of leadership, and of teamwork... It is an account of a hospital where there was a 'club culture'; an imbalance of power, with too much control in the hands of a few individuals.
>
> (*Learning from Bristol*, 2001, synopsis paras 3 and 8)

The Inquiry also saw the need for a major shift in the internal management of the NHS and in particular the development of more open organisations willing to acknowledge and learn from errors. The Inquiry endorsed the recommendations of the Chief Medical Officer's expert group (Department of Health 2000a) designed to create a learning culture in the NHS. It recommended that NHS organisations should identify and learn from sentinel events, 'any unexplained occurrence involving the death or physical or psychological injury, or the risk thereof' (*Learning from Bristol*, 2001: 450).

> Every effort should be made to create an open and non-punitive environment in which it is safe to report and admit sentinel events...Members of staff in the NHS who cover up or do not report a sentinel event may be subject to disciplinary action by their employer of professional body.
> The opportunity should exist to report sentinel events in confidence.
>
> (*Learning from Bristol*, 2001: 450–1)

The Inquiry report reinforced the government's commitment to changing the nature of decision making from one based on clinical autonomy, a system in which professionals relying on professional custom and practice controlled decision making and implicitly assessed and managed risk, to clinical governance, with increased external regulation based on codified knowledge such as guidelines that formed the basis of the explicit formal assessment and management of risk. The aim was to 'restore the trust that society and patients historically had in medicine' (Lugon and Secker-Walker 1999: 1).

Clinical governance represents a major change in management of health care in the UK in which the decisions of individual clinicians are subject to increased external and professional regulation. While clinical governance involves the development of external inspection bodies such as the Commission for Health Improvement, it also involves the development of organisations which can ensure quality and safety. The 1997 White Paper, which established the blueprint for New Labour's NHS reforms, described the ways in which the new 'quality organisations' would identify and manage risk, so minimising harm to patients by ensuring that:

- clinical risk reduction programmes of a high standard are in place
- adverse events are detected, and openly investigated; and the lessons learned promptly applied
- lessons for clinical practice are systematically learned from complaints made by patients
- problems of poor clinical performance are recognised at an early stage and dealt with to prevent harm to patients.

(DH 1997: 47)

Most of these processes can actually be bolted on to existing NHS structures creating new expert hierarchies to audit and manage risk (Power 1997). For example NHS Trusts have created clinical governance committees with responsibility for creating clinical risk reduction programmes, identifying poor clinical performance and reporting results to Trust Boards. However, one area does not fit quite as easily – reporting of errors or adverse events. Within traditional hierarchical bureaucracies the emphasis is on avoiding errors by sanctioning staff who are identified as causing error especially if this involves a breach of rules and procedures. As Hood *et al.* (1992) pointed out, allocating blame creates incentives amongst subordinate staff to conceal errors that result in near misses, that is situations which could have resulted in major disasters; such concealment has been a major factor in man-made disasters such as Bhopal (Turner and Pidgeon 1997). Error reporting implies a significant change in culture and operating procedures as it is based on:

- *A shared value system.* Traditional command and control structures do not require shared values, indeed many classic studies of Fordist production systems indicate very different value systems between managers and operatives (Benyon 1984). In Fordist systems senior executives establish operating rules and procedures and create a supervisory system to ensure that this system is adhered to. Error reporting implies a shared interest and commitment to safety between those providing a service and managers, and a commitment from those delivering the service to identify potential hazards and report incidents;

- *Altruism.* There is no financial reward for reporting an error or a near miss; indeed there are likely to be costs. These will include the time costs of making a phone call or filling in a form and then being party to any subsequent investigation. There is also the possibility that the person reporting an incident may be ostracised by work colleagues and others and blamed and even disciplined by managers. While managers may provide guarantees that those reporting incidents 'in good faith' will not be disciplined, the precise parameters and conditions of such guarantees may not be clear;

- *Partnership.* The emphasis on error reporting as a learning process implies that it is a joint and shared enterprise in which those delivering the service have important and valuable knowledge that they share with senior managers. Thus error reporting is based on a partnership within the organisation based on shared values and trust.

All NHS agencies with a responsibility for delivering services to patients are now expected to have systems to report and monitor adverse clinical events and 'near misses'. In response to the emerging findings of the Bristol Inquiry and to facilitate the development of clinical governance the Secretary of State for Health established an expert group chaired by the Chief Medical Officer, to examine ways in which the NHS could learn from and prevent adverse events. The report of the working group, *An Organisation with a Memory* (DH 2000a), stressed that adverse events in the NHS were often similar in nature to those that occurred in other sectors. The report provided examples of comparable incidents resulting in harm such as 'dangerous omissions' – a failure to replace an engine oil seal in a Royal Flight is compared to the failure to replace partially used containers of intravenous fluid in the NHS (DH 2000a: 43). The working group was particularly impressed by the Aviation Safety System which included mandatory systems for reporting incidents as most of the learning seemed to come from investigation of the nature and pattern of near misses rather than from investigation of fatal incidents (pp. 43–5). The working group recommended that the NHS should create a 'Mandatory reporting scheme for adverse events and specified near misses... rooted in sound standardised local reporting systems' (p. 80). The working party recognised that if this system was to work effectively it would require a change in culture and more of a collaborative approach to development of working practices: 'We recommend that the NHS should encourage a reporting culture amongst its staff which is generally free of blame for the individual reporting error or mistake, and encourage staff to look critically at their own actions and those of their teams' (p. 82). While the working party envisaged a relatively localised reporting scheme with the lessons from each locality being reported to a national local agency, they suggested that, while the necessary system and culture changes were being made, the NHS should create a national system with 'provision for direct, confidential (but not anonymous) reporting' (p. 81).

The Secretary of Health endorsed the main recommendations of the Report in his Foreword (Milburn 2000) and the Department of Health moved rapidly to implement its main findings with two implementation documents: *Building a Safer NHS for Patients* (DH 2001) and *Doing Less Harm* (DH and NPSA 2001). The Department established the National Patients Safety Agency with responsibility for ensuring effective management of risk in the NHS or in NHS-funded care (NPSA 2003). The new agency was designed to improve the quality of patient care by ensuring there are effective systems of reporting, analysing and learning from patient safety incidents, adverse clinical events and near misses. While individual health care providers were expected to create their own reporting systems which are compliant with national standards, the Department agreed to the formation of a national incident reporting and learning system.

The National Patients Safety Agency's role is to improve the safety of patients by promoting a culture of reporting and learning from patient safety incidents within the NHS both at national and at organisational level. The Agency has identified seven steps to improve NHS organisations' patient safety focus. Each NHS organisation should:

1 build a safety culture by encouraging staff to report when things go wrong (look at 'what' has gone wrong rather than 'who')
2 lead and support your staff by establishing a clear patient safety focus throughout the organisation
3 integrate your risk management activity by developing systems and processes to manage your risks and identify and assess things that could go wrong
4 promote reporting by ensuring that staff can report both locally and nationally when things go wrong
5 involve and communicate with patients and the public by developing ways to communicate with them
6 learn and share safety lessons by encouraging staff to analyse the root cause of incidents
7 implement solutions to prevent harm by learning lessons and making changes to practices, processes and systems.

A key feature of the new patient safety strategy is the development of a national error reporting system designed to ensure that staff, patients and carers report adverse clinical incidents and near misses that they are themselves involved in, or which they witness happening (NPSA 2004). Staff who witness or are involved in an incident are expected to complete an incident report form and then information from these forms is aggregated at organisational and national level to identify patterns of incidents, enabling the NHS to introduce preventative action to reduce risk.

The regulatory state is grounded in an inquiry culture which highlights specific dangers and hazards and creates expectations that organisations will identify and effectively manage these risks. In health care, iconic inquiries have highlighted the risks posed by dangerous individuals. Within the NHS such expectations can be linked to the development of a risk or safety culture. An important component of the safety culture is the surveillance system based on the identification and reporting of incidents and near misses which is designed to identify existing and emerging dangers and hazard so that action can be taken to minimise harm and prevent disasters.

Incident and near-miss reporting in the NHS

In the remainder of this chapter we will examine some implications for organisations and their internal relationships of developing incident and near-miss reporting systems. In particular we will focus on why in some contexts such systems do not appear to work as planned and examine why this should be. The data we use in this part of the chapter are derived from a small exploratory study in one National Health Service organisation, a joint NHS and Social Care Trust providing services for vulnerable adults, that is adults with mental illness or learning disability and older people with dementia. We were invited to research the error reporting system in the Trust, because senior managers felt that it was not working well in one part of the Trust. Staff in this part of the Trust did not seem to be reporting incidents. We therefore agreed to focus primarily on areas of low reporting and interview both managers and front-line staff to see how they perceived the system and explore why they felt reporting was low. It is important to stress that this was very much an exploratory study. We were given access to the key policy documents within the Trusts but because of limitations of time and difficulties of access we only conducted nine in-depth interviews – two with managers, one with a psychiatrist, two with clinical psychologists, two with nurses and two with social workers – and another four with front-line staff. Thus our findings need to be confirmed by other studies.

The main drivers for the development of incident reporting in the Trust were clinical governance and the requirement of the National Health Service Litigation Authority, which indemnifies participating NHS Trusts in respect of clinical negligence trusts. Within the Trust the Director of Corporate Affairs acted as the sponsor of the Reporting of Adverse Clinical Events policy and the Trust Board of Directors was actively involved in its development. An early draft was shared with all Executive Directors and some senior managers. The final version was one of over forty policies relating to clinical governance, all of which are accessible to Trust staff through the Trust's intranet. The policy itself was fairly brief. It contained definitions of an adverse event and a near miss (both taken from *An Organisation with a Memory*, DH 2000a) and detailed instructions for the procedure to be followed when reporting an incident or a near miss. It outlined the duty of all staff to report adverse clinical incidents and near misses and it contained a guarantee, signed by the Trust's Chief Executive, that staff would not be blamed for reporting an incident or near miss.

The system was paper-based. Staff who were involved in or witnessed an incident had to complete an incident report form. This form included information about the incident and on the person completing the form, including their name, job title and work telephone number, so that incidents could be followed up by the Clinical Risk Analyst if further information was required. As the system developed so did the complexity of the reporting mechanism. Initially the Trust only required completion of the front page of the incident report form but extended this to include the back page outlining the action taken to deal with the reported hazard and subsequently the Trust introduced a separate form for the reporting of drug errors.

In our interviews with managers and professionals we identified problems with each of the key preconditions for the effective development of an effective reporting system: there was an absence of consensus especially over the framing of issues and the purpose of the reporting system; there was little evidence of altruism, rather there was evidence that reports were used to gain personal or group advantage; and there was little evidence of the development of trust-based partnership replacing command and control hierarchy.

Problems of consensus: framing issues and defining the purpose of error reporting

There was disagreement between managers and professionals who worked with clients about the nature of errors and purpose of the error reporting. Managers saw reporting as objective identification of risks, particularly of 'events or omissions arising during clinical care and causing physical or psychological injury to a patient' (DH 2000a: xiii). This objective approach to risk in which adverse events are treated as 'self-evident' was evident in this manager's definitions:

> The way I see it, [an] adverse event is anything that happens, or nearly happens, and should not have happened. This is, I think, very broad. It's not just about deaths and suicides, it's also about near misses, [and] failures. For example, failure – failure to follow policies, or something that people say they'll do but don't do...anything undesirable, I guess.

In contrast front-line professionals felt that the definition of an adverse event was problematic. It was influenced by professional judgement with different professions using a different framework to define an adverse event. For example a professional with a social care background felt that the Trust's approach was dominated by a health or clinical perspective:

> I think the problem lies with the terminology...because I don't think there's any doubt that, for a lot of social care staff, the term 'clinical' conjures up a health

model. And I think, similarly...with 'clinical' adverse incidents or whatever, the very use of the term 'clinical' kind of...puts a frame in people's minds.

Professionals recognised that even where there was significant harm, for instance when a patient died, it was not self-evident that an adverse event had occurred which required investigation. One front-line professional described the discussion within the team about the nature of one death:

> We have a healthy debate at the moment about whether the death of one of our patients, who is known to our service, but died in the community due to natural causes, should be an SUI [Serious Untoward Incident] or an IRIS [incident report form].

While Trust policy specified that all deaths should be recorded and investigated, professionals felt that some deaths were from 'natural causes' and therefore should not be treated as an adverse clinical event. A professional noted that he did not agree with the decision to treat a death of an older patient as a serious incident as it was from natural causes and that, 'you know, we don't really want to treat every death as though...something went wrong'. Professionals acknowledged the ways in which an adverse event was socially constructed and drew attention to the factors involved in defining an incident within the risk category. One important factor involved external judgements, especially those made by the coroner. For example, one professional saw the coroner as the main arbiter: 'It's up to the coroner to tell us which is suicides and which is deaths [not requiring investigation]...', while another noted: 'If it goes to a coroner, the coroner should indicate whether we need to do an internal inquiry.'

Managers also noted that there was variation in the ways in which front-line staff assessed risks, though they tended to see this failure as a result of skills deficits rather than deliberate oversight or a failure to frame issues in terms of risk. For example, a senior professional in a managerial role using the benefit of hindsight commented:

> When I do a clinical review, after, for example, a suicide, you can see near misses happening along the pathway...but what I'm finding is that people are not reporting those issues, because they don't see them as an 'adverse event'.

Near misses were even more difficult to define and contentious as they did not involve significant harm, as one professional noted: 'There isn't enough clarity about near misses...that's very much more subjective...usually, ninety-nine times out of a hundred, they end up satisfactorily.'

Not only was there lack of consensus on what constituted an incident or near miss which should be reported, but there was also considerable disagreement about the purpose of the reporting system. Managers tended to endorse official trust policy and see reporting as part of organisational learning and development.

One manager emphasised the ways in which information in each individual report created an evidence base for effective risk management:

> Because that's [incident reporting] the only way, at the end of the day, that the Trust is going to know what works and what doesn't, what the trends are, you know, where the service shortfalls are, is if they've got evidence.

Professionals did acknowledge the potential benefits for reporting but tended to see benefits in terms of their professional role and their responsibility for specific clients rather than as general benefits that might accrue to all clients through organisational learning and risk reduction. One professional described a serious incident that she had reported for a number of reasons, the most important of which was 'for the client...because I felt that, if it was reported, maybe someone would intervene, and actually review the situation'.

However, perceived client benefit was in some contexts seen as a reason not to report as the client or patient might suffer as a consequence, especially if the incident involved violence. One professional, who had failed to report an incident where he had been assaulted by a patient, explained why he had not reported the incident: 'I think there is a great reluctance on the part of health professionals to report against patients, because it is part of our care, to tolerate a certain amount of distress in the patient.'

Some front-line professionals were cynical about the purpose of error reporting. They felt it was about organisational rituals and bureaucratic procedures. One noted that 'It's ticking boxes, I think.' While another commented 'That's what they're doing. They're reporting it!' so that the responsibility was transferred up the hierarchy: 'All they need to do is complete these [forms] and senior managers will be told about it.'

Even managers were concerned about the nature of form filling as they felt it prevented professionals from using their skills to effectively analyse and manage risk: 'They're so desperate to fill in the right forms, so they don't get a rap over the knuckles, that they're not using their clinical skills, and they're not reporting the subtleties of risk.' There was a sense in which filling forms had become an end in itself, not a means to enhanced patient care. One professional who had to do risk assessments for mentally ill patients as part of the Care Programme Approach and complete the adverse event reports noted that, 'you know, *that* [form filling] seems to be the care, not the care. The forms have become the care, not the care itself.'

For some professionals form filling was a ritual designed to protect the organisation from blame when things went wrong. Professionals, especially those working within mental health services, felt there were inadequate resources – there was 'massive collusion about how under-resourced we are'. This meant that it was inevitable that things would go wrong, that patients and others would be harmed. One mental health professional described the problems of under-resourcing in the following way: 'We miss some of this...early process stuff...that is basically good practice, that, because people are so stretched, [the work load] does build up, and then we do have these near misses or incidents.' For these professionals, the reporting system was a mechanism for organisational reassurance and a way of deflecting blame when things went wrong:

> I think we're sort of – we *partly* feel better because we've got this, you know, huge mechanism...to capture these things. So, in a way, as an organisation, we feel *better*. But I think, in a way, it's a defence against all these other things, that are bubbling away under the surface.

They did not accept the view that error reporting was about organisational learning, rather they saw it in terms of blame allocation: 'I don't feel that the whole reporting mechanism, and the way it's explained within the Trust, supports a learning culture at all. I think it's – people see it as – pinning the blame.'

Lack of altruism: blame and selection of issues to report

The lack of a sense of shared purpose and a sense of global benefit were not conducive to the development of altruistic motivation in error reporting. This was compounded by cynicism about the no-blame guarantee provided by the Trust's Chief Executive. One professional suggested that 'the Trust's "no-blame" policy is seen as rhetoric, rather than reality'. Some were forthright: 'I don't think it's [the Trust's "no-blame" policy] worth the paper it's written on, really.' Another was equally sceptical: 'People *know* "no-blame" doesn't work, because people *will* always be to blame.' Professionals felt that, while the Trust claimed that the error reporting was blame free, the actual process of investigation did not convey the same message. A social worker professional described the process in the following way:

> You know, almost straight away, you get this sort of feeling, of well, you know, 'they've taken our files' and 'they're scrutinising them' – but they're saying it's 'blame free'. That's a hard one. It's really hard.

There was a perception that if a serious incident occurred then the emphasis would be on blame: 'If it's something trivial, you'll get off, and people will say, "Hey, we're a 'no-blame' culture." But if it's a serious incident, somebody will be hung out to dry.'

Some professionals contrasted the formal reporting system which exposed staff involved to investigation and blame with informal systems that provided protection: 'My experience is that there are mechanisms where my colleagues feel free to come and tell me...it's done in an atmosphere where – it's done confidentially, protecting the person. That's my experience, anyway.' A number of professionals, while acknowledging the limitations of the no-blame guarantee, did not see the fault as lying within the Trust, rather they felt senior Trust Executives and Directors were reflecting external pressure and the fear of being the subject to a major disaster and inquiry: 'It's the national blame, I think, that worries people, more than the internal blame. I think we constantly work under this fear of doing something that's going to become a national inquiry.'

Altruism is an important component of error reporting because staff will only report all errors if they are confident that it will contribute to a general good, otherwise they will be selective, only reporting errors when it serves their purpose. The professionals in our study indicated that they are selective in their reporting. They felt there was a personal cost in reporting both in their own exposure to potential blame but also because it could threaten their relationship with their work colleagues. Most front-line staff felt that individuals avoided reporting because they felt it undermined their position, especially their membership of informal groups. One professional described reporting as 'taboogenic' (sic) and 'like a violation of something, and you're crossing a boundary. There is a built-in resistance, to violate an unwritten law, or a code, or a boundary...to transgress.' Another professional felt that 'People get very defensive, working in a team. It's about "snitching" and all that stuff.'

Thus professionals felt that individuals reported incidents to protect themselves, especially when they felt they had no other option:

> That's what it feels like. It's like – they'll find a way of *not* reporting because they feel it will expose them. Or they feel they absolutely *have* to report, because they might, you know, something might befall them... But if – and this is a really difficult thing to talk about – but my sense is that people use reporting to protect themselves, one way or another.

Another noted that individuals made reports to ensure that 'the blame isn't pinned on them'. Some professional staff noted that they used the reporting mechanism to cover themselves where disagreements occurred within multidisciplinary teams, or where they felt that they might be blamed for someone else's action (or inaction). For example a professional who felt that reporting was 'like snitching' reported an incident when there was a professional conflict and difference of opinion over the discharge of a patient to ensure his position was clearly documented if anything happened.

Issues of fairness and ownership

Underpinning the official rhetoric is an emphasis of shared learning and partnership in reporting. Partnerships are essentially egalitarian and to operate effectively depend on members feeling that they are fairly treated, otherwise they will withdraw their cooperation. Front-line professionals, especially lower status professionals such as nurses and social workers, did not see the reporting system as fair. They felt that staff groups could use their status and power to avoid reporting incidents and any associated blame. There was a shared perception that medical staff did not report incidents:

I've never seen an IRIS [incident reporting] form completed by a medic, ever, or a psychologist, I don't think...either they don't know about it, which I find very surprising...or they don't see it as their job... I've had this before, in another incident...I told [the doctor] that I needed an incident form. He instructed the ward staff to do it!

Non-medical professionals noted that doctors did not even acknowledge drug errors and that when they made such errors simply rectified them:

Doctors frequently prescribe incorrectly, or don't date entries, or give wrong doses. The nurse will bring it to their attention, and it'll be changed. But in theory, that's an IRIS reporting incident, but it doesn't happen. They just correct it.

Even managers acknowledged that doctors did not comply with error reporting requirements. One manager noted that 'the medics are very comfortable with the risks they manage' and another stated that nurses did most of the reporting while 'doctors are the weak link in our risk analysis'.

Front-line staff perceived the system to be unfair not only in differential reporting but also in differential blame. They felt that both personal and professional factors influenced who got blamed. One front-line professional drew attention to personal factors:

Then it comes down to popularity. If you like them, and they're usually a good bloke, and you think they've probably had this one-off mistake, they might get off. But if it is someone they wanted to get rid of anyway...their feet won't touch the floor.

Professional factors were seen as important, with nurses and social workers attracting more rapid and stronger sanctions than doctors. For example one nurse noted that if a nurse was blamed then that nurse would be rapidly disciplined, whereas it took far longer to discipline doctors and they were often exonerated:

I mean, looking at the medical suspensions, nationally, nobody ever seems to know how to manage a doctor's suspension, even though, to everyone else, they look like open and shut cases. And there's two years' suspension, and then, quite often, reinstatement. Or somebody moves to another job.

A front-line professional recollected a specific incident in the Trust in the following way: 'I mean, the nurse was done and out within a month, but the consultant...a year on, they're still deciding...who'd hear it, and who'd be on the panel, and all those sorts of things.'

The lack of fairness of the system related to professionals' perceptions that they did not own the system. It was not a partnership but an imposed system and therefore an extension of hierarchical relations. One professional who asked not to be quoted on this issue clearly saw the reporting system as imposed from the top while another who was less reticent stated: 'I mean, this is a very driven reporting culture. It's a very "top down" [in the] Trust, not "bottom up".' The managers we interviewed felt that there had been consultation over the implementation of the error reporting system. For example one manager when asked about consultation said: 'I've not been involved, but reasonable. I would say the ownership's reasonable. I mean, it gets discussed at clinical governance, there's a level of consultation that you've been through...' However, when we explored exactly who had been involved, it became clear that it was mainly senior managers, especially those involved in clinical governance. One manager commented: 'It's unlikely that all staff down there will have seen the draft, but it certainly went to the senior management', while another who was a member of the Clinical Governance Committee noted: 'I think within governance [that is, the Clinical Governance Committee] we were reasonably consulted about how it's developed. We've changed it about six times!'

The absence of partnership meant that several of the front-line professionals saw the main purpose of error reporting not as improving patient care by reducing errors but protecting the Trust from external sanction. They felt pressure to report selectively by not reporting on issues which might expose the Trust to criticism. One front-line professional when asked about the organisational learning potential of error reporting commented:

> Because we're trying to protect the Trust from litigation, we're not as open and honest about the facts of things as we could be. ... [We put] a sort of sub-conscious or unconscious slant [on things]... There's a lot of – how can I put it? – 'Oh yes, well, but this explains that, so we won't get into that, will we?' sort of thing.

While another noted: 'I think a lot of staff, if they're going to keep something quiet, it's because they want to keep it quiet internally. It's more they are worried about external influences.'

Front-line professionals saw the error reporting system as one part of an overall strategy to protect the Trust from risk and blame including the proactive management of the Trust's media image. For example in a discussion of a high profile incident in a neighbouring Trust which attracted adverse media comment and criticism, a front-line professional commented:

> We're a very press-conscious Trust and I think it just helps, if you're 'press aware'. I mean, in [a nearby Trust], for example, they get a lot of hostile press, even though they seem to be one step ahead of things.

Conclusion

Both social scientists and government ministers tend to see the current concerns about risk as a product of increased anxiety amongst citizens about the uncertainties of living in late modern society. For example Taylor-Gooby has drawn attention to the paradox of timid prosperity in which increased security is associated with increased anxiety:

> Material levels of security in the western world are higher than ever before... However, the sources of uncertainty and the mechanisms available to most people to deal with them have changed, leading to the paradox of timid prosperity – growing uncertainty amid rising affluence.
>
> (Taylor-Gooby 2000: 3)

The government acknowledges that a modernised high-trust public service (DH 2000a, para 6.1) should protect individuals not only from harm but also the anxieties associated with potential harm, whether these are the fear of crime, terrorist attack or a pandemic of avian flu. Its dominant approach to increasing public confidence and trust is to increase regulation and the use of encoded knowledge, indicating that it no longer trusts key NHS staff, especially doctors, to use their own judgement.

As Bradach and Eccles (1989) note, collaboration is based on transactions (the exchange of goods, services or knowledge) which can be managed in different ways, such as through markets, authority or trust. Transactions are usually facilitated by a combination of two or three of these methods, though typically one is predominant. Thus, in the NHS, collaboration is based on authority combined with elements of markets and trust. This provides for both strong regulation and integration and close ties between high status individuals (Goodwin *et al.* 2004: 60) but does not facilitate the broader participation, voluntary cooperation and shared identity (Goodwin *et al.* 2004: 33) required in a partnership such as the one envisaged by the error reporting system. If the health care system is to develop an effective system for 'organisational learning' then it must find a better balance between authority and trust based on effective communication 'in terms of teamwork as networks have been seen to work most effectively where there is freedom of decision making and an ongoing shift from explicit to tacit knowledge and *vice versa*' (Castells 2000: 169–71).

Such an approach may help managers in managing risk. Currently they are only a near miss away from a disaster and inquiry. With an increasingly hostile media, a culture of inquiries, legal principles such as vicarious liability and corporate manslaughter plus the development of hyper-innovative policy making senior managers are increasingly vulnerable. Actions that they have little awareness of or control over can have major consequences for their reputation and livelihood. While the managers in our study were committed to and believed in a reporting system as a way of identifying and managing risk, they recognised that they needed the cooperation of key professional staff, especially of medical staff. They needed to create a shift in power so that the self-regulatory club culture of doctors was subject to the external regulation. There was in this exploratory study little evidence of a fundamental shift in power. While professionals such as nurses and social workers were aware of and made conscious decisions whether or not to treat a specific incident as a near miss, doctors appeared to remain aloof and did not see the system as applying to their decisions. Recognising and acknowledging the intuitive knowledge of professionals is central to demonstrating that they are trusted and without such demonstration they will undermine systems which depend on their active cooperation.

References

Beck, U. (1992) *Risk Society: Towards a New Modernity.* London: Sage.

Benyon, H. (1984) *Working for Ford.* Harmondsworth: Penguin.

Bradach, J. and Eccles, R. (1989) 'Price, authority and trust: From ideal types to plural forms', *Annual Review of Sociology* 15: 97–118.

Burgess, A. (2006) 'The making of the risk-centred society and the limits of risk research', *Health, Risk and Society* 8: 329–42.

Castells, M. (2000) *The Rise of the Network Society.* Volume One (2nd edn). Oxford: Blackwell.

Department of Health (1997) *The New NHS, Modern Dependable*, Cm 3807. London: The Stationery Office.

Department of Health (2000a) *An Organisation with a Memory: Report of an Expert Group on Learning from Adverse Events in the NHS.* London: The Stationery Office.

Department of Health (2000b) *The NHS Plan*, Cm 4818-I. London: The Stationery Office.

Department of Health (2001) *Building a Safer NHS for Patients: Implementing an Organisation with a Memory*. London: The Stationery Office.

Department of Health and National Patient Safety Agency (2001) *Doing Less Harm.* London: The Stationery Office.

Department of Health and Social Security (1982) *Child Abuse: A Study of Inquiry Reports, 1973–1981.* London: HMSO.

Giddens, A. (1991) *The Consequences of Modernity.* Cambridge: Polity Press.

Goodwin, N., 6, P., Peck, E., Freeman, T. and Posaner, R. (2004) *Managing Across Diverse Networks of Care: Lessons from Other Sectors.* HSMC Services Management Centre, University of Birmingham.

Green, J. (1997) *Risk and Misfortune: The Social Construction of Accidents.* London: UCL Press.

Heyman, B. (2004) Editorial: 'Risk and mental health', *Health, Risk and Society* 6: 297–305.

Hood, C.C., Jones, D.K.C., Pidgeon, N.F., Turner, B.A. and Gibson, R. (1992) 'Risk management', in The Royal Society Study Group (eds) *Risk: Analysis, Perception and Management.* London: The Royal Society.

Kemshall, H. (2002) *Risk, Social Policy and Welfare.* Buckingham: Open University Press.

Learning from Bristol: The Report of the Public Inquiry into Children's Heart Surgery at the Bristol Royal Infirmary 1984–1995 (2001) Command Paper: CM 5207. London: The Stationery Office.

Lugon, M. and Secker-Walker, J. (1999) Introduction, in M. Lugon and J. Secker-Walker (eds) *Clinical Governance: Making it Happen*. London: The Royal Society of Medicine Press, pp. 1–5.

Lupton, D. (1999) *Risk*. London: Routledge.

Milburn, A. (2000) Foreword, in Department of Health, *An Organisation with a Memory Report of an Expert Group on Learning from Adverse Events in the NHS*. London: The Stationery Office, pp. v–vi.

Moran, M. (2003) *The British Regulatory State: High Modernism and Hyper-Innovation*. Oxford: Oxford University Press.

National Patient Safety Agency (2003) *National Reporting and Learning Systems*. Available at http://www.npsa.nhs.uk/health/reporting/background (accessed March 2007).

National Patient Safety Agency (2004) *Seven Steps to Patient Safety: An Overview Guide for NHS Staff* (2nd print). Available at http://www.npsa.nhs.uk/health/resources/7steps (accessed August 2007).

Power, M. (1997) *The Audit Society: Rituals of Verification*. Oxford: Oxford University Press.

Report of the Inquiry into the Care and Treatment of Christopher Clunis (1994). London: HMSO.

Rothstein, H. (2006) Editorial: 'The institutional origins of risk: A new agenda for risk research', *Health, Risk and Society* 8(3): 215–21.

Smith, R. (1998) 'All changed, changed utterly', *BMJ* 316: 1917–18.

Taylor-Gooby, P. (2000) 'Risk and welfare', in P. Taylor-Gooby (ed.) *Risk, Trust and Welfare*. London: Macmillan.

Turner, B.A. and Pidgeon, N.E. (1997) *Man-Made Disasters*. Oxford: Butterworth-Heinemann.

Chapter 6

Ecological validity and risk management in forensic mental health services

Jacqueline Davies, Paul Godin, Bob Heyman,
Lisa Reynolds and Monica Shaw

> Bad or Mad: The conviction of another psychiatric patient for manslaughter and attempted murder once again highlights a failure to protect either the public or the patient themselves from serious harm... He [the offender] now faces indefinite incarceration under the Mental Health Act.
>
> (BBC 2006)

The above radio report referred to the outcome of attacks by a mental health service user in December 2004. The report blames services for not predicting the risk of offending. In this chapter we will argue that the task of risk assessment in this context raises inherent difficulties. We employ the concept of ecological validity as an analytic tool to consider the difficult task of risk assessment for discharging service users from forensic mental health services.

As with many other areas of health care delivery, forensic mental health care services have to contend with the risk management dilemma of balancing safety against patient autonomy and freedom. Forensic mental health care aims to protect a vulnerable society from a group of vulnerable service users whose behaviour has been recognised to be a serious threat to public safety, whilst affording them freedom and autonomy in their rehabilitation back into the community. In this chapter, we chart some of the practices of what Rose (1998) describes as 'risk thinking', the pervasive discourse and practices of risk assessment and risk management that have come to characterise contemporary mental health care, and particularly forensic mental health care (Heyman *et al.* 2004).

We explain the concept of 'ecological validity', drawn from the arena of social science experiments, which we apply as an analytical tool to understand risk thinking within forensic mental health care. We will draw on data from a four-year qualitative study of an English medium-secure unit to explore how risk thinking has made the experience of the forensic service user like that of a subject in a social science laboratory experiment undergoing a battery of tests and close observations. The concept of ecological validity both helps understand the processes of risk assessment and risk management of service users. As they move through from the high to low risk levels of the forensic mental health care system, the concept sheds a new light on the behaviour of forensic mental health service users and their more or less strategic responses to being the objects of risk assessment. Patient responses to risk assessment are little researched or understood and are to date still conceptualised in terms of adaptation to institutional life (Goffman 1961).

Ecological validity's contribution to sociological thinking about mental health care

Goffman's mid-twentieth century classic study of total institutions explored how psychiatric patients adapted to the demands of the asylum system. After more than a century of continuing growth it was then more overcrowded than it ever had been before and was heading into inexorable demise. Goffman described how inmates developed primary and secondary adjustments to accommodate demands for institutional efficiency and conformity, which eroded individual autonomy leading to the mortification of the self. He showed that patients were in a dilemma. In order to get discharged they needed to conform. Yet in doing so they lost their ability to act autonomously. Applying the concept of ecological validity to the critical analysis of forensic mental health services could be dismissed as a mere recycling of the critique of institutionalisation offered by Goffman in *Asylums*. However, at the time that Goffman wrote about institutionalisation, the world, including mental health care, was very different from now. Then psychiatric in-patients were expected to conform to the regulatory discipline of the long established unchanging order of the asylum system. They were required to relinquish their civil self to become mental patients subject to block treatment. Now that the asylum system has been dismantled mental health patients are, as Castel (1991) asserts, profiled and re-profiled through risk assessments from which they are assigned social trajectories to follow as they are risk managed towards an optimum state of functioning. Thus in the secure mental hospitals of the forensic mental health care system, patients are continually assessed and processed individually towards their rehabilitation. Mental health patients are now not so much expected to relinquish selfhood to conform to the demand of the psychiatric system but are rather expected to develop themselves as responsibilised individuals.

Forensic mental health care developed in its modern form from the building of medium and low secure units to replace the lunatic asylums for the criminally insane (now called high secure special hospitals). Forensic care is the one area of contemporary mental health that has considerable similarity to the old asylums. Like the asylums, forensic units and special hospitals accommodate mental health patients for long periods of time on a compulsory basis. However, mental health care radically transformed itself in the latter part of the twentieth century with a substantial move towards community care, not only in the UK and in the USA (from where Goffman gathered most of his data for *Asylums*) but, with some variability, in almost all advanced industrial nations (Goodwin 1997). Rose (1996) described the change in marine geographical terms with the asylums depicted as submerged land, leaving a complex system of psychiatric archipelago in a sea of community care. Features, other than the location of care, may be identified with the transformation of mental health care, such as a shift from a focus on mental illness to mental health and more generalised practices of mental health care (Rose 1990). Perhaps of greatest significance has been the development of risk thinking, a development that Castel (1991) identifies as part of a long-term trend away from thinking about mental health service users as dangerous, towards a population-based reasoning about the risks that mental illness poses, producing the 'epidemiological clinic'. Practitioners and policy administrators have developed elaborate technologies and strategies of risk assessment and management to manage service users along individually planned paths of care towards their optimum functioning.

However, this highly rational world of risk assessment and risk management is far from a well-ordered bureaucracy. Forensic mental health care is beset with inherent problems, ironies and deceptions (bluff and double bluff). In order for those detained as forensic service users to be released they are required to redeem themselves from their 'high risk' status, ascribed to them on the grounds that they are offenders with mental health problems and that such offenders are more likely to transgress in the future. However, the ecology of such units differs substantially from the outside world, making risk assessment inherently problematic. We argue that this problem corresponds to that of ecological validity in the classical social psychological experiment discussed by Orne (1962) and Orne and Holland (1968). Both in laboratory experiments and risk assessments in secure units, there are differences between the controlled environment where observations are made and the outside world where conclusions are applied. Orne noted the influence of social-psychological dynamics on the behaviour of subjects in social science research who sought to please their experimenter, and the impact of laboratory-based deceptions devised to access supposedly psychological information. Forensic mental health service users seek to please their clinicians in the hope of gaining autonomy. Similarly the clinicians engage in deceptions in the hope of finding (again) supposedly true psychological information on which risk assessment can be based. In the heyday of asylums, staff stripped patients of their selfhood, through denying their civil identities and destroying their autonomy (Goffman 1961). Now staff seek to get to the core of the patient by other means, such as deception, to achieve conformity of a different sort. For staff who take a psychodynamic approach, deception is readily available to them in the toolkit of their discipline. One psychoanalytically oriented psychiatrist told us that a crucial skill in psychoanalysis was using deception to access the unconscious mind. Others may use deception on the same groups as the experimental social psychologists of the 1960s, in order to penetrate the mask of self-presentation and uncover the true level of risk which patients pose.

The inmates of the asylums studied by Goffman in the 1950s were not subjected to constant risk assessment as they are today. Forensic mental health patients in the twenty-first century are intensely and continually assessed so that their risk status can be measured. Orne's concepts of ecological validity become particularly apposite. Martin Orne developed the concept of ecological validity to critique conclusions about obedience and conformity drawn from laboratory experiments by the social psychologist Stephen Milgram. Orne's concept of ecological validity encompassed three observations. First, that subject behaviour in the artificial conditions of a laboratory experiment cannot be generalised to daily life. Second, subjects actively respond to the 'demand characteristics' of experiments, by which the subjects tried to understand the purpose of the experiment. Third, subjects responded to the demand characteristics by attempting to comply with or subvert the experiment. These last two issues were dealt with in the classic psychology experiments by deceiving subjects about the purpose of the research.

Unlike Goffman's inmates, medium secure unit (MSU) service users are closely observed in an artificial environment to assess their level of risk. Below we will first describe some of the history that has led to changes in forensic mental health care. We will then discuss how risk assessment and management in forensic mental health care has made the experience of a service user in a MSU like that of a subject in a social science laboratory experiment with reference to a study in one such unit.

The history of risk management in forensic mental health care leading to the clinic as a social science laboratory

In the 1960s selected patients were discharged from secure settings, first in the USA (Steadman and Cocozza 1974) and then in the UK (Prins 1999). This policy was motivated by concern for the autonomy of the individual (Tidmarsh 2002). The subsequent reoffending by some of these individuals (particularly Graham Young, discussed below) highlighted the problem of assessing patients in high secure (special) hospitals for living in the community (Prins 1999).

Graham Young was discharged from a special hospital under a policy to rehabilitate mentally disordered offenders. He was sent to Broadmoor in 1962 for poisoning members of his family. Fourteen years later he was discharged, and killed work colleagues, drawing upon the poisoning skills which he had developed in the high security hospital library (Prins 1999: 238). Prins points out that 'although there was (rightly) concentration upon his [Young's] education needs, perhaps not enough attention was paid to his emotions and continuing preoccupations with poisons and killing'. In Broadmoor, Young studied medical texts, improving his knowledge about the effects of poisons on the human body. With hindsight, the ecology of the special hospital had provided opportunities to observe Young's preoccupation with poisons and killing, but within that ecology his studies were supported as desirable educational activities. To make the point clear, Prins compares Young to a violent offender who may win praise for his involvement in body-building classes whilst in prison when another view might be that he was keeping himself fit for further mayhem upon discharge. The pressure to be occupied in hospital, regardless of how inappropriate the activity might be for long-term development, arises in the context of managing a group of potentially volatile individuals who must live closely confined together with little opportunity for leave. This is summed up in a quote from a service user involved in a qualitative study in an Australian forensic secure facility: 'Well, when you've got up to 25 people living together in one locked up unit, sooner or later sparks are going to fly. If anyone expects anything else they should be locked up in here with us!' (Meehan *et al*. 2006: 21).

In the light of the Graham Young case, a report by the Committee on Mentally Disordered Offenders recommended the establishment of regional secure units (Home Office and DHSS 1975) to create a more appropriate setting to assess and identify the service user's propensity to reoffend than that provided in the remote locations and esoteric environments of high secure (special) hospitals. The development of MSUs was reinforced by a further report (DoH/Home Office 1994) which more explicitly spelt out the advantage of a halfway setting where patients could be observed and assessed in an environment closer to community living than special hospitals.

The problems of employing actuarial risk management techniques were discussed in the first Home Office report: 'actuarial prediction methods can identify high-risk and low-risk groups, [but] they will always leave a residual majority in "middle-risk" groups, whose rates are too near "fifty–fifty" to be of much use' (Home Office and DHSS 1975: 60). Despite this caution note, statistical techniques, similar to those used in social science laboratory experiments, have become a central feature of forensic mental health risk assessment. Actuarial tools based on epidemiological studies of offending behaviour are used in risk assessments. (One such tool, the HCR-20, will be discussed below.)

Formal risk assessment

While informal assessment and clinical judgement may be based largely on current behaviour, formal tools such as the HCR-20 put more emphasis on the historical events than any others (see Table 6.1). The HCR-20, a twenty-item inventory, asks ten questions about the history (H) of the service user, five about their current clinical (C) state and a further five about their future risk management (R). In the second version of the HCR-20 published in 1997, the authors (Webster, Douglas, Eaves and Hart) explain that they devised the tool in 1994 for their own practical purposes and were surprised by the widespread international interest which it generated. The status of high risk is ascribed on the grounds that previous offenders are more likely to transgress in the future. This is reflected in half the items being based on the service user's history. However, this history cannot be altered therapeutically to reduce a service user's risk status. Anyone with a high score on the basis of previous behaviour will have difficulty escaping from their high risk status.

Table 6.1 Risk assessment domains covered by the HCR-20

Historical	Clinical	Risk management
H1 Previous violence	C1 Lack of insight	R1 Plans lack feasibility
H2 Young age at first violent incident	C2 Negative attitude	R2 Exposure to destabilisers
H3 Relationship instability	C3 Active symptom of major mental illness	R3 Lack of personal support
H4 Employment problems	C4 Impulsivity	R4 Non-compliance with remediation attempts
H5 Substance use problems	C5 Unresponsive to treatment	R5 Stress
H6 Major mental illness		
H7 Psychopathy		
H8 Early maladjustment		
H9 Personality disorder		
H10 Prior supervision failure		

The main mission of MSUs, the safe rehabilitation of patients into the community, can only be achieved through bringing about changes in the non-historical areas which somehow 'override' the historical indicators. Meeting this requirement demands heavy reliance on assessment of the clinical and risk management items listed in Table 6.1 above.

The ecological validity of risk assessment in MSUs

We draw upon a qualitative study of risk assessment in a medium secure unit to illustrate how forensic services must manage ecological validity problems in assessing whether a service user can be moved towards greater autonomy and lower risk management. Since 2001, we have undertaken research into risk assessment and management and rehabilitation in an English MSU. The study was designed to explore the processes of risk assessment and management through which mentally disordered offenders progress across levels of secure settings until they are deemed safe enough to return to the community (DoH 1999).

Over the time we have visited the MSU the difference between the unit and the outside world has increased with a gradual increase in security measures. In line with the 2000 Department of Health Report, the site, like all MSUs, is now surrounded by high chain fences, creating a surreal visual contrast with the community-oriented architectural style of the original buildings. The climate has shifted away from a focus on rehabilitation to an emphasis on public safety, undermining the normalcy which they were intended to promote.

The MSU was described by a general manager as 'a step-down unit from high secure hospitals and a step-up service from PICUs (Psychiatric Intensive Care Units) [locked wards in general psychiatric services]'. The MSU had a series of wards from intensive care, where only plastic cutlery and cups were allowed and limited contact was permitted beyond the confines of the ward; through a range of wards where access continued to be controlled through electronic and physical barriers with increasing opportunities to leave the ward; to 'Rehab' (rehabilitation) where service users prepared their own food (with metal knives), and eventually were granted progressively longer periods of escorted and then unescorted leave into the community. However, we argue that no matter how gradual the progression from secure to communal living, the nature of the risk management process leaves the service user in a role similar to a classic psychology subject. Predictions about their behaviour in the community are derived from observations of what they do in a very different ecology.

Our research started with an induction to the MSU including safety training and visiting all the wards and concluded with feedback seminars with staff. Throughout these stages we built an understanding of how service users were assessed through hypothesis testing and a trial and error approach of giving service users greater autonomy, for example through access to potentially dangerous tools such as knives and a graded system of leave from wards and the MSU. Clinicians predicted what might happen and then observed what did happen. Service users undergoing these assessments sometimes 'second guessed' the intentions of the staff. For example, one man described how his psychiatrist alternately said he would recover completely from his mental illness and that he would be on medication for the rest of his life. The service user believed the psychiatrist did this to provoke him into anger. However, the service user never asked his clinicians if this was the case. In turn the staff engage in deceptions to control for the service users' attempts to speed their release by complying with therapeutic programmes, and admitting to 'insight' and 'remorse' as required by their carers and the instruments with which they are tested. The emergent theme of service user and provider experience being like subject and researcher in a laboratory emerged from the beginning of the research.

In our first round of research interviews we spoke to 45 staff members. In the second round, we developed profiles of ten service users based on interviews with them and the staff involved in their care, with informed consent. During the analysis, all participants were given pseudonyms and these will be used below. In our analysis of interviews we adopted the term 'ecological validity' when discussing the intractable problem of how to assess the risk of a service user reoffending in this esoteric environment.

Among the anonymous examples given by staff and the ten profiled service users we came across men and women with a range of problems (Davies *et al.* 2006). In this chapter we will focus on how service users and their problems are validated differently by clinicians. At one extreme there was Boyd who sought the safety of living in a hospital environment, partly because it kept him away from children and other vulnerable members of the society whom he had a history of offending. His strategies for living peacefully in the MSU included an 'anamnestic' solution of waking up very early, and being asleep when most service users were enjoying free time in the evening. At the other extreme, Noel found it difficult to live in a communal ward without getting into fights both with staff and fellow service users. While Noel anticipated that he would offend less away from the close confines and authoritarian rules of the hospital, his discharge seemed to become ever more distant each time he was involved in a violent incident on the ward.

We argue that secure environments offer poor ecological validity for predicting the post-discharge behaviour of the two service users described above. For those whose offending involved targets not present in the unit, hospital was a sanctuary where daily living problems were managed, temptation was removed and there were few triggers for offending. While such service users were easy to manage on a daily basis and made rapid progress towards low security, finding suitable tests with which to assess them for discharge was difficult. For others whose offending had involved violent arguments with peers or rebellion against authority the unit was a pressure cooker in which they repeatedly exploded with rage and returned to the intensive treatment unit. While these individuals were described by service providers as having anger management problems, the Australian study referred to above (Meehan *et al.* 2006) suggests that the MSU is a pressurised environment in which anyone would find it difficult to live peacefully.

Service users and service providers who participated in the study said progress through the high to low risk hierarchy of wards was dependent on being unproblematic to manage on a daily basis on a previous ward (Heyman *et al.* 2004). In that article we argued that this did not mean that those who did not cause trouble were more fit to be discharged than other service users, but such a move might start the service user on a trajectory towards a (possibly) unwarranted discharge. One ironic contrast we observed was that those who are so keen to return to the community that they abscond find themselves further from discharge, whereas those who are content to live in the institution move through the system towards discharge. The latter group were largely those whose offending histories were untested within the secure setting and therefore most difficult to ultimately discharge. Because of the difficulty in predicting what might happen after discharge from the ecology of the unit, the decision to discharge was difficult to make and service users could spend a long time in the low secure wards. Service providers used informal and formal risk assessment measures to try and balance the process of rehabilitation, and one of the tools most frequently mentioned was the HCR-20 (discussed above).

The study revealed a number of recurrent themes around the problem of ecological validity generated by the artificial conditions in the MSU. These include the demand characteristics of living in the environment and the primary and secondary adjustments made by patients to manage their lives. The findings begin with an illustration of the contrasting views of a senior and junior staff member. The manager presents an organisation that is blind to issues of ecological validity whereas front-line staff must cope with such issues on a daily basis. Second, the data analysis offered below will be concerned with how the demand characteristics of an MSU's ecology may prevent patients from offending or provoke patients into offending. Third, the data analysis shows how the patients manage, or fail to manage, the demand characteristics through compliance or subversion. Some continued with behaviour from their culture of origin which was perceived as inappropriate in the MSU. However, a high level of compliance by patients was treated as suspicious by staff.

Staff awareness of ecological validity issues

The general manager of an MSU presented the aims of the unit without apparent reflection on the ecological validity of predicting future offending from within the unit.

> We should take somebody who has committed an offence while they have been unwell. Bring them in here and be able to, it could be that it is homicide, but bring them in here and treat them and be able to put them back in the community somewhere around eighteen months to two years.
>
> (George, general manager)

The two-year period referred to above was prescribed by the 1992 Department of Health Report. This measured period seems realistic in the unproblematic process based on a disease model of treating mental disorder presented above. In George's view, the service user's disorder can be removed from the individual. He shows no concern for how the staff will assess the risk of the service user reoffending in the community. While the above manager showed apparent disregard for ecological validity, front-line staff were often acutely aware of differences between the hospital and external environments. In contrast a health care assistant on a rehabilitation ward said of her colleagues: 'you are dealing with forensic patients. But there, over here I think a lot of the staff sort of forget that...generally they've had sort of settled patients' (Paula, health care assistant). Paula used the term 'settled' which harks back to the idea of institutionalisation. While they may have learnt to live harmoniously with staff on the ward, they may not have developed skills that prepared them for the challenges of rehabilitation and preparation for discharge. Similarly, a nurse who participated in our study of a South African forensic hospital (Reynolds 2006) observed that just because a service user does not steal in hospital where there is nothing to steal does not mean that he will not steal after he has been released.

Prevention from reoffending

In the interviews, staff were asked to give anonymous examples of cases that had progressed more or less well. One case that most closely fitted the model given by George (above) was described by a psychologist. She described a man who had killed his child in a drug induced psychosis:

[He] came in here [MSU] and he recovered very quickly from this psychosis, really within days. He was well at the time he came to us, but of course very, very depressed for a long time, partly reactive to what he'd done but I think there was some evidence that he was depressed before that, but actually quite ready to, to leave the unit after a year, after [a] relatively short period of time.

(Pamela, psychologist)

Despite (in Pamela's view) being ready, this service user was not discharged until some time later. Pamela suggested that this was because he was being 'punished' by some staff for his offences. However, there was no way of knowing how this man would behave after discharge, and the indicators of reduced risk which he provided, such as showing remorse, might have been displayed in order to lower his risk status and thereby secure earlier release. As we developed profiles of service users who participated in our study we became aware of others who were seen as good service users while on locked wards but for whom discharge was seen as dangerous. We met Malak on the rehabilitation ward. He prayed five times a day, kept himself clean, went to his classes and always took his medicine. Despite presenting few management problems on the ward, the staff were concerned that he might harm his family once discharged but they had no way of checking this out while he was on the ward. Similarly, a profile service user who likened himself to the biblical character of Daniel in a lion's den could not obviously be assessed. He had learnt to cook and went to church but the risk of him returning to his past offending pattern of sexually assaulting girls once he was discharged could not be tested. Both Malak and Daniel were held in the low secure unit awaiting discharge while staff puzzled over how to safely assess the risk of discharging these service users.

Provocation into reoffending

Unlike the men described above, others were assessed as high risk because of the problems which they caused whilst living at the MSU. A social worker described a discharged service user who stayed in the MSU for years because

[Alan's] personality was such that he would be hostile and would go back into [a] higher level of security... It was safe [to discharge him, but] incredibly difficult for an in-service team to present a care plan to community colleagues to say that mental health is now in remission, but what is left is a personality type which is basically antisocial.

(Patrick, social worker)

According to the social worker, the service user's response to the ecology of constant observation and communal living led to him being 'confined in a spiral' leading to 'rebellion and pushing against the structure'. However, he won his tribunal and was discharged into the community where he makes a living as a writer and can avoid communal living and hierarchical situations. His case can be compared to that of a caged animal who behaves atypically in a zoo. In both cases, behaviour in one atypical ecology does not provide a reliable guide to behaviour in another. Although the social worker felt certain that the service user could be safely discharged, a judgement which from the perspective of hindsight proved correct, it is difficult to identify the grounds for his confidence. In effect, he discounted the problems which this patient presented in the ecology of the MSU, reasoning about how he would behave in a community environment.

The MSU service user quoted below had been moved to a higher level of security in response to a chain of events which he depicted as follows:

> I was told [my friend] was dead. And that made me upset, and I was crying for the whole day. Then, the next day, I got up, I wanted to go to the shops to get hold of my, you know, washing my clothes and stuff, and just getting over it, you know, and, um, they [ward staff] wouldn't let me go out. They made my life hard... This member of staff, he actually called the [Emergency Response Team], and they are there specifically to inject you with something to knock you out. Now, I didn't want to be knocked out, not after my friend died, and I didn't want to go through any grief. So, I just lost my temper and I smashed up [the ward].
>
> (Noel, profile service user)

The chain of events begins according to his own account with the service user grieving in response to the death of a friend. This normal, culturally validated, response is treated as pathological, triggering compulsory medication which, in turn, impels him to respond violently, and then causes him to be moved to a higher level of security, re-acquiring a higher risk status. However, from the service user's perspective, the first cause of this incident was the untherapeutic staff response to his grief. According to him, his angry response therefore had low ecological validity in relation to his conduct after discharge. For the purposes of this chapter, it is not necessary to endorse any individual's perspective. Our aim is to illustrate the interrelationship between the problems of risk assessment and ecological validity. Staff working at the MSU tended to understand the behavioural problems of service users in terms of institutionalisation. A nurse manager talked about 'jailing behaviour', and a nurse consultant saw outbursts against authority which ended in a backwards move towards higher security as 'gate fever' designed to avoid the anxiety associated with discharge. Noel's behaviour could represent secondary adjustment to institutionalisation subconsciously designed to avoid discharge, as suggested by staff. However, it could equally well involve a response to the demand characteristics of a very difficult situation. Orne (1981) might have described Noel's response as the 'screw you effect' and that Noel was refusing to participate in a process designed by the clinicians.

Demand characteristics: behaviour in context

The following example illustrates the way in which social action which would be considered acceptable in one social context could be interpreted as an indicator of riskiness in another. William's consultant regarded his money-making practices, such as providing a hair cutting service for other service users, as an indicator of his high risk status. However, William saw himself as a local lad whose behaviour was misunderstood in the MSU, but would be perfectly acceptable in his community of origin, the East End of London, with its long tradition of small-scale and sometimes dubious entrepreneurial activity. Service users could experience the minute observation of their behaviour within a 'forensic' framework of meaning as oppressive.

> Well, about for instance. I walked across to the table, the pool table, tapped on the top of it, and she [the nurse] wrote down that I was feeling aggressive, and that, and all things like that. And I just thought, well one tap on the table. I thought that was entirely wrong. So I said. She discussed it. It came out in the ward round. That. She wrote that, which was wrong, out of order.
>
> (William, profile service user)

All clinical nurses are expected to observe service users throughout the day and night and write notes. These notes are later interpreted by a clinical team, often without the presence of the nurse who wrote the notes. Service users soon learn that notes are written about them outside clinical meetings, and that these notes are interpreted for clinical purposes. Like research subjects, service users reflect on how they present themselves and how their behaviour is interpreted. What happens in the MSU is influenced by the dual meaning of the term 'forensic' in this care context, encompassing both serious crime and a reassuring but problematic sense of precision. However, nurses and others undertaking risk assessments have to undertake complex interpretations of what they happen to observe, as illustrated by the following quotation about a service user whose responses to stress were seen as too good to be true:

> There was this issue about his girlfriend getting married. You know, he wasn't happy about it that his family never told him that [she was] getting married. Apart from that every time Stan [said] 'Oh, I'm fine. I'm alright', you know. 'Have you got anything you are worried about?' 'No', you know. He's no worry. We can't be 100% sure, but, oh, 'Stan is well. Stan is fine', you know. We obviously have to be cautious because you never know what might happen, you know, and that's why we need to monitor his mental state really closely. He's all pleasant, he's normal, and it's alright, but you never know what will happen, you know. So we [are] just keeping a close eye on that. We know he's the 'star service user' and everything. But we have to watch him, given that what he did before, you know, and how he did it.
>
> (Leticia, Stan's primary nurse)

Because of his offending history, Stan would have scored as at high risk on the H (history) component of the HCR-20, the standardised questionnaire used to assess risk, and therefore needed to achieve a very low score on the other two elements (C, current clinical, and R, future risk). The primary nurse was concerned that Stan was playing an information game (Goffman 1953) with the intention of lowering his risk status. In terms of ecological validity, Stan, according to the nurse quoted above, understood the demand characteristics of the situation, but had not appreciated that those assessing him would question his impression management.

As well as possibly 'faking good behaviour' in order to improve their release prospects, or at least being viewed as attempting to do so, service users could adopt remarkably complex and non-obvious strategies designed to achieve personal short-term objectives. The service user discussed below had apparently faked serious forensic mental health symptoms in order to be granted supervised leave:

> He [Boyd] said that he wanted to rape someone, he wanted to abscond, he wanted to hurt a child. And they still let him go because he turned round and said, 'Well I made it all up. I just wanted to go and see my mum'... I would not escort him.
>
> (Isobel, health care assistant)

In effect, this service user may have faked high risk status in order to be judged ill by medical staff who controlled most decision making and invoke a therapeutic response. In the above case, this complicated ploy succeeded as Boyd was granted escorted leave.

With respect to the central case of service users seeking to speed their release as much as possible, staff may give service users tacit or explicit clues about what is required of them in order to reduce their risk status. Nevertheless, some may fail to understand the message. The service user quoted below had resided in secure settings for over 20 years:

> And the nurse told us quite frankly that this is the gateway, the doorway to freedom, you know. That's what she said. And I appreciated that, you know. Afterwards, I thought it was fantastic that she said that. I never [heard] anybody else say it before, you know.
>
> (Tom, profile service user)

This approach may be understood as 'hinting' to patients who had not, over a long period of time, grasped the underlying demand characteristics of the situation. It stands in contrast to deceptive tactics designed to catch patients out in order to uncover concealed riskiness. These two tactics, taken together, reflect the contradiction inherent in the forensic mental health care task, namely enabling rehabilitation and preventing reoffending. Tom's explanation of what he had been told about the gateway may be interpreted in the frame of ecological validity that he had been advised to follow the demand characteristics of the forensic situation:

Well I suppose I played the game the right way, you know. I mean, I was here and I play the game the right way, that's to keep quiet and wait, you know, to get better.

(Tom, profile service user)

This last quotation, from a staff perspective, generalises the reframing of the therapeutic process as acceptance of demand characteristics:

Service users get worn down really... It's not really that you become all that better. You've just accepted what's going on, and you just say, 'This is my lot. I'm going to do my time and get on with it there'... This settled thing that people are talking about, I think, is just a case of getting used to the environment or the rules and regulations.

(Kunle, charge nurse)

Reducing service user riskiness to a level acceptable for their release, reframed in terms of them accepting the unit regime, raises the question of the ecological validity of conformity as an indicator of reduced risk status, just the question which was asked about Stan, 'the star patient', as discussed above. Service users who wished to speed their release needed to manage a delicate balancing act designed to avoid being accused of overacting or of rebellion.

Conclusion and discussion

In this chapter, we have compared the problem of assessing the risks posed by forensic mental health service users to that of making valid inferences from classical psychology experiments. Research subjects engaged with the demand characteristics of classical psychological experiments involving deception, demonstrating a tendency to seek to control their destiny in the face of manipulation. Equally, forensic mental health service users may seek to affect their progress through the system. However, for service users the information game they undertake with those observing and assessing them is much more important than it is for participants in a time-limited psychological experiment.

Service users spend time in a 'secure' environment designed to minimise the risk of them harming themselves or others. Depending upon the nature of their previous offences, its ecology may conceal or exaggerate their apparent propensity to reoffend. Both service users and staff may, depending upon their degree of reflective awareness, attempt to take into account the demand characteristics of the risk assessment situation, creating more or less complex and reactive information games.

The value of social science laboratory experiments was challenged by Cook and Campbell (1979) when they recommended quasi-experimental design in field settings. Observing service users while in community care is difficult, and the resulting risk assessments are criticised when low frequency, high impact incidents occur. Quasi-experiments therefore provide a very difficult model for forensic mental health risk assessment. While MSUs were first intended by the Home Office to provide quasi-community settings, the impact of recent UK Department of Health measures designed to increase security levels at MSUs has been to make them even less like the environments which discharged patients return to than were the original MSUs. This reversal of the intended plan for forensic units has led to the increase in stages at the lower end of security and the extension of time which service users spend in the secure settings. Along with the increased focus on risk management, greater security has led to forensic units being more like the laboratory settings studied by Orne than the asylums studied by Goffman.

Instead of viewing themselves as operating a culture of care, clinicians are now involved in supposedly objective observations and risk measurement, using 'instruments' which are claimed to accurately predict the risks posed by individuals. Some service users perceive this shift with suspicion, and may see themselves as engaged in information games rather than a therapeutic relationship (Godin 2006). Service users may attempt, or may be accused of attempting, to conceal their 'true' risk status. However, many become frustrated because they fail to speed up their discharge, and become caught in the system, as illustrated above. The strategic or other responses of service users to being the objects of risk assessment are little researched or understood.

Although our data cannot document the factors associated with length of detention, our research suggests that those whose offences possessed low ecological validity in the medium secure environment, for example child sex offenders, at least had available to them the option of attempting to pass through the system without the issues which led to them offending being addressed. However, unless they presented evidence of their risk status with some subtlety, they risked losing their credibility. Arguably, an optimum strategy for achieving early release might involve displaying gradual conversion to accepting the legitimacy of the service regime after an initial period of resistance intended to demonstrate that the service user was not merely pretending to be a 'star patient'. At the other end of the spectrum, some service users constantly cycled round the wards as they struggled to manage the frustration of living with constant observation and other techniques for their risk assessment and management. In contrast, for patients with presenting problems, such as Noel quoted above, the frustrating environment of the MSU had high salience. Arguably, at least, if he could control his anger in the MSU he could contain it elsewhere. His failures or refusals to do so repeatedly set him back. However, as illustrated by the case of Alan, discussed above, such patients may prove capable of controlling their anger in the less constraining environment they would return to after release. In consequence, some service users may remain in secure settings because they cannot control their anger there whilst they would, if released, be acceptably low risk in a less stressful environment.

The shift to the epidemiological clinic identified by Castel (1991) has brought the process of risk management closer to the experimental laboratory where predictions are based on assessed probabilities. The critique of the classical social psychological experiment can usefully be applied to the problem of risk assessment in forensic mental health service contexts. In both cases, inferences about behaviour in one social context are derived from observations of behaviour in another, raising the question of ecological validity. In our study of risk management in the MSU we concluded that this shift towards risk thinking has altered the behaviour of both clinicians and service users which reflect what was observed with the studies of ecological validity. It is argued that pressure to improve risk management in mental health care has put health care outcomes for patients in second place (Holloway 1996; Petch 2001).

In this chapter, we have focused on the case of mentally disordered offenders cared for in forensic mental health medium secure units. But the issue of ecological validity could equally be applied to risk assessment and management for other service users who may appear to learn to manage their health problems in hospital, but may be ill-prepared to manage these problems when they return home, for example those who are shown how to use complex medication processes (for example injections) in hospital but must manage without daily clinical help at home.

References

BBC (2006) Onlinebbc.co.uk/London 11/8/06 (Kurt Barling report) http://www.bbc.co.uk/london/content/articles/2006/03/06/mad_bad_feature.shtml (accessed June 2007).

Castel, R. (1991) 'From dangerousness to risk', in G. Burchell, C. Gordon and P. Miller (eds) *The Foucault Effect: Studies in Governmentality*. London: Harvester Wheatsheaf, 281–98.

Cook, T. and Campbell, D. (1979) *Quasi-Experimentation: Design and Analysis Issues for Field Settings*. Boston, MA: Houghton Mifflin Company.

Davies, J., Heyman, B., Godin, P., Shaw, M. and Reynolds, L. (2006) 'The problems of offenders with mental disorders: A plurality of perspectives within a single mental health care organisation', *Social Science and Medicine* 63: 1097–1108.

Department of Health (1992) *Report of the Working Group on Psychopathic Disorder.* London: Home Office, Department of Health.

Department of Health/Home Office (1994) *Report of the Working Group on Psychopathic Disorder.* London: Department of Health/Home Office (Reed Report).

Department of Health (1999) *National Service Framework for Mental Health*. London: Department of Health.

Department of Health (2000) *Report of the Review of Security at the High Security Hospitals*. London: Department of Health.

Godin, P. (2006) 'Engaging service users in the evaluation and development of forensic mental health care services', fmh website. Available at http://www.nfmhp.org.uk/Godin%20final%20report%20to%20website.doc (accessed June 2007).

Goffman, E. (1953) *Communication Conduct in an Island Community*. PhD dissertation, Department of Sociology, University of Chicago.

Goffman, E. (1961) *Asylums: Essays on the Social Situation of Mental Patients and Other Inmates*. New York: Anchor Books, Doubleday and Co.

Goodwin, S. (1997) *Comparative Mental Health Policy: From Institutional to Community Care*. London: Sage.

Heyman, B., Shaw, M., Davies, J., Godin, P. and Reynolds, L. (2004) 'Forensic mental health services as a health risk escalator: A case study of ideals and practice', in B. Heyman (ed.) Special edition on Risk and Mental Health. *Health, Risk and Society* 6: 307–25.

Holloway, F. (1996) 'Community psychiatric care: From libertarianism to coercion. "Moral panic" and mental health policy in Britain', *Health Care Analysis* 5: 235–43.

Home Office and DHSS (1975) *Report of the Committee on Mentally Abnormal Offenders* (Butler Report). CM 6244. London: HMSO.

Meehan, T., McIntosh, W. and Bergen, H. (2006) 'Aggressive behaviour in the high-secure forensic setting: The perceptions of patients', *Journal of Psychiatric and Mental Health Nursing* 13: 19–25.

Orne, M. (1962) 'On the social psychology of the psychological experiment with particular reference to demand characteristics and their implications', *American Psychologist* 17: 776–83.

Orne, M. (1981) 'The significance of unwitting cues for experimental outcomes: Toward a pragmatic approach', *Annals of the New York Academy of Sciences* 364: 152–9.

Orne, M. and Holland, C. (1968) 'On the ecological validity of laboratory deceptions', *International Journal of Psychiatry* 6: 282–93.

Petch, E. (2001) 'Risk management in UK mental health services', *Psychiatric Bulletin* 25: 203–5.

Prins, H. (1999) *Offenders, Deviants or Patients?* London: Routledge.

Reynolds, L. (2006) 'Travelling down the risk escalator: A qualitative study of forensic mental health services in South Africa', 6th Annual International Association of Forensic Mental Health Services (IAFMHS) Conference.

Rose, N. (1990) *Governing the Soul*. London: Routledge.

Rose, N. (1996) 'Psychiatry as a political science: Advanced liberalism and the administration of risk', *History of Human Sciences* 9(2): 1–23.

Rose, N. (1998) 'Living dangerously: Risk-thinking and risk management in mental health care', *Mental Health Care* 1(8): 263–6.

Steadman, H. and Cocozza, J. (1974) *Careers of the Criminally Insane: Excessive Social Control of Deviance*. Lexington: Lexington Books.

Tidmarsh, D. (2002) 'The level of risk posed in care of the mentally disordered offender in the community', in A. Buchanan (ed.) *Care of the Mentally Disordered Offender in the Community*. Oxford: Oxford University Press.

Webster, C., Douglas, K., Eaves, D. and Hart, S. (1997) *HCR-20: Assessing Risk for Violence (Version 2)*. Burnaby, BC: Mental Health Law and Policy Institute, Simon Fraser University.

Chapter 7

Talking and taking risks

An exploration of women's perceptions of antenatal testing in pregnancy

Dawn S. Jones

It has become almost clichéd in sociology over the past few decades to pronounce the social world as increasingly characterised by a plethora of choices, possible decisions, and potentially risk-laden scenarios. The phenomenon of pregnancy is no exception (Katz-Rothman 1994), and represents a key site through which the connections between health, risk and vulnerability can be demonstrated. Indeed, as with other chapters in the book, the politics of health, risk and vulnerability emerge as integral to this research, allowing an insight into how discourses of risk work to shape and govern the ways in which pregnancy is defined and treated.

In this chapter, I explore how women receive 'high risk' screening results during pregnancy, and how they discursively communicate with other women about risk. In other words, I am investigating the relation between 'objective', medically defined assessments of risk, and 'subjective' or emotional responses *to* risk, by the women in my sample. Exploring discourses from an Internet discussion forum, a number of key questions are raised. How do narratives that look at 'high risk' antenatal screening results in pregnancy contribute (or not) to 'objective', scientifically validated perceptions of risk? In other words, what is the 'fit' between 'objective' 'expert intrusions' into the body, and 'subjective' 'lay' forms of knowledge about risk? (Beck, in Beck and Willms 2004). And how – if at all – can talking about 'high risk' results amongst pregnant women destabilise medical narratives of such risks? Additionally, does 'talking through' risk increase or decrease the levels of vulnerability and anxiety that women face when receiving a 'high risk' screening result from health care providers? When labelled as either at 'high' or 'low' risk of having a baby with 'abnormalities', what effect does such a classification have on women's emotional stability and sense of well-being? In exploring the politics of risk transmission, from health care provider to 'consumer', the significance of the language of risk for one's sense of security is key to how risks are perceived. While Douglas (1986) has suggested that institutional classifications can lead to a situation in which subjects appear to lose independence over their perception of a situation, placing them in a position of existential vulnerability, my research throws up a number of emerging themes that appear to challenge a simplistic top-down model of risk transmission and reception.

To summarise the main points of my argument, my findings suggest that the label 'high risk' in the context of health care provision in pregnancy creates a subject whose sense of security is threatened. In talking through risk with other potentially vulnerable individuals, a variety of discursive 'coping strategies' are, however, in evidence, suggesting that, while vulnerable, the 'at-risk' self can negotiate, and even challenge, the objective classifications of risk made by health care providers. Whether attempts to destabilise medical definitions of risk by subjects can be seen as a threat to the status of antenatal testing and the values and interests of the National Health Service is, however, questionable.

Having outlined the main focus of my chapter, the discussion will now turn to address the theoretical context in which my research might be understood. In looking at the approaches of writers such as Ulrich Beck and Anthony Giddens, I explore how a theoretical approach to risk testing might be developed. I then go on to consider the methods and methodological context of my research, addressing specifically the use of covert research methods in the collection of my data. An outline of the method of critical discourse analysis then follows, and a discussion of the themes and issues surrounding Internet text analysis is provided. Having presented extracts from the discussion forums studied, I then attempt to relate my emerging findings to a broader discussion on how antenatal testing in pregnancy might be understood in relation to themes of health, risk and vulnerability. Finally, I make some conclusions, and provide a reflexive account of my role as researcher.

Theoretical context

Theoretically, my research draws upon and contributes to the tradition of risk analysis developed by Ulrich Beck through his writings on what he has termed 'risk society' (1992; Beck and Willms 2004). The position I take, and the arguments that I make here, are broadly supportive of Beck's analysis of 'risk' as a systematic way of coping with uncertainties and insecurities created and developed by modernisation itself (Beck, in Beck and Willms 2004: 21). Relating this rather abstract statement to the area of health and the 'at risk' self, a number of points can be made. First, it can be claimed that the development of antenatal testing itself, and the growth of research into scientifically 'improved' ways of calculating the health of the foetus in pregnancy, can be seen as an attempt to 'govern the ungovernable': that is, to monitor and take action to screen 'at risk' pregnancies so as to identify those which may need to be 'managed'. As such, the growth of research to develop more accurate, 'objective' screening, so as to identify early on in pregnancy 'abnormal' foetuses, can be seen as a way of coping with the vulnerability of both scientist and health care provider in the face of naturally occurring medical conditions. In a quest for 'ontological security', risk testing can thus be considered, à la Beck, to be symptomatic not only of a fear of the unknown, but of the political, economic and cultural implications that might stem from failing to identify 'high risk' pregnancies.[1] As Beck has argued, 'risks depend on decisions, that are industrially produced and in this sense politically reflexive' (1992: 183). Both Giddens' and Beck's approaches to science in late/new modernity are useful, examining how risk is reduced to probabilities, and hence open to calculation and rationalisation by the scientific community. And yet, while scientific research continues in its search for certainty and future benefits, the traditional dichotomy between expert and layperson has, according to Beck, been transcended by the rise of reflexive modernisation (Beck *et al.* 1994). Scientific discourses become unstable, challenged as they are by the critique of expert opinions from, for instance, citizens, the media, and even within science itself (Giddens 1990). And yet, simultaneously, the vulnerability and insecurity that such a critique creates for both scientist and layperson does itself create a greater need *than ever before* for certainties and securities, though now the decisions about how to deal with such 'risks' are very much left to individuals. This is not to say that science has given way to other expert discourses. To quote from Beck on this, the fear and insecurity that is present in the new modernity has meant that we 'end up with a world in which it is impossible not to make decisions, and it is impossible not to make them based on scientific reasoning' (Beck, in Beck and Willms 2004: 203). When looking at the topic of antenatal testing in pregnancy, Beck's analysis is suggestive of a climate in which women's anxiety and uncertainty about the risks they face in pregnancy reflect precisely the dilemmas that reflexive modernisation create. Such tests might thus be seen as reflecting a vulnerable community of scientists, health care practitioners, and politicians, facing the 'risk' of the perceived increase in economic, political and social 'costs' that children with disabilities might be associated with. Furthermore, in attempting to regulate risk through antenatal screening programmes, Beck's perspective draws attention to the consequences of such testing procedures on women and their partners. To some extent, the uncertainties that risk testing throws up is, as Beck suggests, a consequence of attempts in late modernity to 'manufacture' risk, with the vulnerable subject constructed *through* such tests, and not as in any way existing prior to entering into such programmes. While testing is entirely voluntary, as Beck has suggested, discourses of risk, and the consequences that follow if one is labelled as at 'high' risk of carrying a foetus that may have 'abnormalities', may create a space in which screening is considered a rational and reasonable course of action. That the vulnerable self exists alongside such seemingly rational actions is, as Beck suggests, one of the many contradictory consequences of late modernity, reflective of how the objective and subjective dimensions of health risk coexist in paradoxical ways. It is this relation between objective and subjective risk, expert and layperson, the institution and social actor, that I wish to explore here, looking at the range of strategies that actors use to 'deal' – in a context of insecurity – with the risks that science 'throws up'.

Method and methodology

My research was conducted through the method of covert participant observation in an Internet antenatal 'club', directed at women whose babies were all due in the same month. Being pregnant at the time myself (and 'due' in the same month as others in the stream), I was able to immerse myself in day-to-day chat, without having in any way to 'pretend' to share the same concerns as those being voiced, yet I did not at any point reveal my academic interest. In other words, the fact that I was researching women's perceptions of risk in pregnancy was not revealed, though no other details about myself, my job, family and personal details were fabricated (at least, not for the purpose of research!).[2] I discuss the ethical dilemma that choosing to remain covert in my method created in the following section.

I visited and posted regularly on the site (at least daily), and used a pseudonym (as all posters do). The other posters in my sample ranged in age from late teens to early 40s, with occupations ranging from 'stay-at-home mums' (SAHMs) to professionals (the latter dominating). The majority of women were pregnant for the first time, closely followed by second-time mothers, then those pregnant for the third and fourth time. All but one poster were having 'singleton' pregnancies[3] (the one exception being a twin pregnancy). I reflect later, in the reflexive section, on the ambiguous position that I, as a pregnant researcher, found myself in when partaking in Internet chat, over a number of months, with women with whom I seemed to share so much in common.[4]

The topic of conversation that I have selected for analysis in this chapter relates to a discussion surrounding one poster's antenatal screening results. The screening programme carried out here is the 'integrated test', which combines blood work with a nuchal fold ultrasound scan, to give a 'risk calculation', in this case, of carrying a foetus with Down's syndrome.[5] The 'cut-off' point for classification of results as indicating a 'high risk' of chromosome abnormality is greater than 1 in 250, with anything above 250 considered a 'low risk' of having an affected pregnancy. The case considered here relates to a 1:2 result, and the subsequent anxiety and uncertainty that this generates.

Covert research: a reflection

The research method that I have selected is covert participant observation. The fact that my research is covert, with the participants unaware that their discussion is part of my analysis of risk in pregnancy, carries with it a number of methodological considerations, not least the ethical dilemmas that such a research method throws up. In making such a decision, I have had to balance the obtaining of informed consent from research subjects against the desire to obtain knowledge that might otherwise have been presented differently (Herrera 1999). While I do believe that when contemplating engaging in covert research the researcher must fully consider the moral and ethical consequences of his or her research on the unwitting participants, I do nonetheless believe that the environment in which my research was conducted (i.e. the Internet) does in many ways negate the ethical dilemmas facing covert researchers in 'real life' environments such as the 'gang' or religious 'cults'. As Howard (1993) argues, public discussions on the Internet are, for many researchers, considered 'fair game' for analysis. The Internet is a public forum, with the discussion analysed here freely accessible to anyone with Internet access. As Norris has argued 'it is common practice to consider anything posted to any list or newsgroup as public information, although one should be cautious that no-one is harmed' (1994). In other words, I suggest that in participating in publicly accessible online discussions one in some way forfeits the right to privacy. In gaining online attention from others, with relatively little effort, one loses simultaneously the control that one may appear to have in 'real life' over how others 'use' what we choose to reveal to them in conversations and discussions.[6] 'Consent' to be researched becomes, for some researchers, of decreasing relevance when the data that is to be utilised already 'pre-exists' the inception of the research project (Hewson *et al.* 2003). Bordia (1996) also suggests that providing the covert researcher ensures confidentiality, and the participants are fully aware that their postings are within the public domain, then the approach does not raise ethical problems.

From a purely pragmatic point of view, it could also be argued that requesting consent might in itself 'skew' the validity of the data with, for example, participants 'withholding' certain thoughts and opinions, or even withdrawing completely from the discussion forum. As Douglas (1986: 4) has argued, 'secrecy is a necessary requisite to obtaining knowledge from possible relevant sources'. In other words, I suggest that, while I have not been 'open' with the research participants through keeping the purpose of my interventions in the discussion forum 'hidden', I would suggest that this in no way constitutes a form of moral or ethical 'deceit'.

Furthermore, as discussed below, Internet discussions are, by their very nature, unpredictable and constantly shifting in form and direction. To have attempted to obtain consent from subjects from the start would, in my opinion, have potentially affected the frankness with which the discussion was conducted. However, on a practical level, the 'open' nature of Internet forum discussions, where anyone is free to enter and leave, would have created difficulties in keeping track of participants with whom to ask consent. As Homan (1991) has argued, covert research such as this is not, I believe, necessarily harmful to participants, with those who enter such discussions in 'cyberspace' already aware that pseudonyms are used, and that care must be taken not to put up personal details such as telephone numbers and email addresses (though many do). Indeed, it could be argued, as many have done (Herrera 1999; Grinyer 2002), that overt, open research, in which informed consent from research participants is obtained, does itself frequently avoid fully explaining research procedures, often has to persuade people to be part of the research, and even uses additional, non-consented data such as research diaries to record observations about subjects (Homan 1991). Indeed, as I claim in the reflexive section of this chapter, I believe that the covert nature of my research has impacted more negatively upon me than upon those who have unwittingly become the subject of my research.

Nonetheless, this is by no means to suggest that research ethics are of no concern. In line with research guidelines by the British Sociological Association, I have safeguarded the anonymity of the research participants by using pseudonyms and by concealing the Internet source used.

For a detailed discussion of the themes and issues relating to the use of Internet discourse as an object of analysis, please see the section on discourse analysis.

The following section reproduces extracts of text from my pregnancy discussion forum. For reasons of brevity, I have had to edit the full discussion, but have selected what I consider to be the key contributions from the 'moment of crisis' that is considered here.[7] Note that any grammatical/spelling errors/abbreviations are reproduced, and squared brackets used to add my own information where considered necessary. While pseudonyms were used by posters, I have changed these to protect the 'net identities' of those who have posted here.

Extract from Internet pregnancy discussion forum, May 2005

Jenny: Hosp just called to say my integrated test shows a 1:2 chance of DS [Down's syndrome]. I'm very worried and upset.

Alice: Oh Jenny, you must be very worried, are you going to opt for amnio? [Amniocentesis]. I'm sure it'll be OK [smiley face].

Tania: Jenny – hopefully everything will be fine and maybe the others can shed some light on this subject. I know nothing as usual.

Debbie: Please don't panic. I had a high risk screen (with first daughter) and had amino as well...all turned out well. I don't think that they stress enough that these tests are 'screening tests' and that for some women 'abnormal' results are normal patterns of bloods for them...for every 100 women who screen for Downs Syndrome, 20 will come back as high risk. Of these 20, 1 to 2 will actually have an 'affected' baby, the other 18/19 will be fine.

Zoë: Jenny just wanted to let you know that a friend of mine went through this but everything turned out OK, so please keep your spirits up. Will be thinking about you tomorrow.

Jenny: Thanks Debbie – the information you posted has helped. I just don't know what to think. Have an appointment with obstetrician tomorrow morning. Any more advice of Qs to ask would be very welcome – my head is reeling!

Tina: sorry about the news Jenny. Please try to keep in mind this is not a definite (diagnostic test) and they are often wrong. I had a high for spina bifida with dd [dearest daughter] and it was wrong she is fine!! My only advice as a s/midwife [senior midwife] and parent is think very carefully about having an amnio (this sounds harsh I know) as there is not much point having one if you would not consider termination; the only advantage to it would be you would know about the condition before birth. If you do have an amnio FISH [fluorescence in situ hybridisation] is great; we normally get results back in 4 days considerably better than 3 weeks. Sorry if this sounded harsh (don't mean to upset anyone) remember most babies are perfectly healthy even after a high result.
Thinking of you tina.

Becky: Jenny sorry to hear your news you must be frantic...I think what Tina has said is very important too as sometimes we may just know too much information which can make making hard decisions even more difficult.

Jenny: thanks for support. DP [dearest partner] and I freaking out a bit.
1 in 2 chance is really very high. Phone call came completely out of the blue following bloods given on Thursday (I thought nothing of it, having had two nuchals a private combined test which gave a result of 1 in 7000) this one was an nhs [National Health Service] integrated test. I really wasn't expecting any bad news at all.
I understand the logic of thinking very carefully before having an amnio but I really don't think I have a choice. Could any of you just wait and see which side the coin lands?
Spent the whole of the afternoon and evening feeling v. [sad face], I cry if I think about termination (seems so ugly, cruel) and I cry if I think about the duty and the idea of not having the baby I imagined.
Tommorow's scan can only be bad/worse or neutral. I feel only getting good results with amnio can make things right again.

Alice: jenny, sorry didn't mean to sound like its an easy decision to make, just be aware of the risks as I had a friend who had the same result and had an amnio but baby was fine, but the procedure didn't go to plan and she lost her baby girl, she obviously felt devastated as there was nothing wrong with her baby. I'm not sure weather [sic] I should have wrote that, as I don't want to scare you and the risk is quite small – don't quote me but I think it 1–2% risk of m/c [miscarriage] from procedure.
At the end of the day, it's you and your partner's decision, make sure you both talk it through, talk with the consultant and ask him as many Q's as you can, best of luck+love xx

Jenny: 99% that amnio won't cause miscarriage vs. 50% baby may have DS. What a mindf**k. anyhow stop researching and go to bed – don't want to be tired and emotional tomorrow. Bye all.

Tina: Jenny will be thinking of you today. I remember clearly how traumatic it was to have a midwife turn up on my front door at 4pm on a Fri. night to tell me about the high neural tube reading, it felt like the world had ended. Try and stay positive as your nuchal readings were excellent. One question is to ask how many amnios does the consultant perform a month/year?? The more they perform the lower the rate of miscarriage for patients generally (it drops as low as 0.5%)
Anyway let us know what happens all my love tina.

Jenny: just back from hosp. taking rest of day off. Consultant was very nice. Scan did not show any DS markers at all...so that lifted our spirits a bit...anyway will get ultimate answer on Friday. Still worried and upset. Dp and I both up and down, tearful then buoyant. Now starting to think we may continue whatever, as we can't bear thought of stopping his/her life having seen him/her again on screen. Anyway, if we do get through this without a miscarriage we are going to find out the gender. Life is too short. Fingers crossed...
[4 days later...]

Jenny: I feel dreadful, still no news, crap sleep, adrenaline rushing through my body, I'm shaking, I have butterflies, I feel sick, I have diahorreah type feelings in my gut, headache, heartache. Dp and I shared a bath this morning before work, and just cried and cried and cried. I don't know what we will decide/do if it comes back positive...

Jenny: [row of smiley faces]
We are very very lucky indeed. After a good weep of relief, we can't stop grinning at each other [row of smiley faces]. Thank you all very very much for caring about us.

Jenny: a 1:2 risk!!!! How lucky are we that this baby is okay?

Discourse analysis of extract: textual strategies, emerging themes, and potential effects

Following Fairclough's (1992) three-dimensional procedure for conducting critical discourse analysis (CDA), this part of the chapter examines the notion of risk at three levels: an analysis of textual features ('description'), emerging themes (meso-level interpretation), and how the text can be understood as a social practice (macro-level explanation) reflecting, and potentially affecting, the social world. As Fairclough himself has claimed, the level of detail and procedures selected by the analyst will very much depend on the discourse type and research agenda; furthermore, it is not uncommon that there will be overlap between each section of analysis. Bearing this in mind I have been selective in the features I wish to examine, looking specifically at discursive features which illustrate best the ways in which women 'receive' and communicate risk in pregnancy.

Description

In this section I am concerned to point out some of the discursive strategies used by posters, looking at features such as choice of vocabulary, tone (modality), politeness mechanisms, and presence or absence of power hierarchy. While all the features identified here point to the development of certain perceptions of risk by posters, with textual features conveying a certain impression of the 'reality' of receiving a 'high risk' antenatal screening result, this section is primarily concerned to describe, rather than interpret, the features so identified.

Choice of vocabulary

The language used by posters is informal and chatty, encouraging a good degree of emotional openness and intimacy with fellow posters. *Choice of vocabulary* such as 'Oh Jenny'; 'it'll be OK'; 'will be thinking about you'; 'are you going to opt for amnio?' contribute to a communicative environment that invites participation, with a sense of togetherness, camaraderie even, amongst a community that would appear fragmented outside of the discussion forum (Jones 1995). The *use of metaphor* is also a dominant feature of the discourse, perhaps suggestive of the need to put into simple, understandable terms a range of complex feelings and responses. For example, the following metaphorical phrases are present: 'maybe the others can *shed some light*'; 'keep your spirits up'; 'my head is reeling!'; 'out of the blue'; 'see which side the coin lands?'; 'lifted our spirits'; 'at the end of the day'.

A further striking feature of the discourse is the use of what Fairclough terms *politeness strategies* and *repair mechanisms* (1992: 163). As Murray (1996) argues, such discursive practices are a 'useful way of gaining insight into social relations', with posters often keen to defuse any potential for misunderstanding that might exist. There are also examples of 'prophylactic repair', where misunderstandings are forestalled through language, again suggesting that the language of risk found here embodies a possible range of highly emotive, potentially upsetting and offensive discourses.[8] Examples of politeness strategies and repair mechanisms include the following: '*hopefully* everything will be OK'; 'Please don't panic'; 'just wanted to let you know'; 'sorry about the news'; 'sorry if this sounded harsh'; 'this sounds harsh I know'; 'sorry didn't mean to sound like its an easy decision to make, just be aware of the risks' (in response to 'flame': 'could any of you just wait and see which side the coin lands?'); 'I'm not sure weather [sic] I should have wrote that'; 'best of luck+love xx'.

Another form of 'repair' – prophylactic or otherwise – is found in the use of emotional symbols ('emoticons' or 'smileys'), used here by the poster to reinforce the spirit in which the post is to be taken. For example, after writing 'I'm sure it'll be OK' in post 1, Alice adds a smiley face, perhaps for added reassurance after asking what might be seen as a possibly intrusive question, 'are you going to opt for amnio?'. The final posting in the discussion is framed by a row of smiley faces, before any written text, declaring, in a fanfare-like gesture, the exuberance felt by the good news received. A further row is also included mid-text, with other grammatical features such as liberal use of exclamation marks, and word repetition ('Thank you all *very very* much') contributing further to the highly excited emotional state of the poster.

The overall tone or modality of the discourse suggests a close, emotionally intimate group, anxious to convey their empathy with 'Jenny' in coming to terms with her 'high risk' result. The next section starts to focus on the 'meso' level, examining the styles of discourse, the 'preferred meaning(s)' of the text, and the ways in which understandings about 'risk' are constructed and communicated through language.

Interpretation

In this section, I start to consider the *relation between* text and context, examining the knowledges that posters bring to the practice of discursive communication, and how the text's 'preferred meaning' is developed by genres of knowledge that exist outside of the text (Baym 1998). To examine first the styles of discourse, or 'genres', contained within the text, a number of observations can be made. First, while the discourse might be classified, at first glance, as 'discussion', or 'chat', there are also more specific 'types' of discourse: for example, requests for information. The most striking styles of communication relate to the frequent citing of *anecdotal knowledge*, combined at times with knowledge about medical/scientific procedures. For instance, Debbie and Tina both merge personal stories with a more detached rationalisation of the 'risk' through the inclusion of medical, scientific knowledge. Debbie's admission that she has been through a similar experience is followed up with statistics which challenge the validity of the risk calculation that has been received in the first place [post 4]. Similarly, Tina's posts combine factual statement with personal experience. The potential effect is to create a degree of empathy and intimacy with Jenny, through having shared to some extent the experience of being told that one had a 'high risk' pregnancy, while at the same time attempting to look 'beyond' the vulnerability of the self through a rational, non-emotive discussion about medical knowledge. It may be adduced that the intention of posters is to reassure through a range of knowledge types and discursive strategies, being involved enough to 'care', and yet able to present the 'bigger picture' of what is at stake when negotiating and challenging the risk as it has been presented by the screening programme ['Please try to keep in mind this is not a definite (diagnostic test) and they are often wrong']. It is interesting that Tina's knowledge as a midwife places her in an ambiguous subject position, belonging both to the medical community that conducts such, apparently 'flawed', tests on a daily basis ['we normally get results back in 4 days...'] and to the community of the 'parent', only too aware that, from her own experience of screening, such tests give out 'wrong' results.

Where posters do not openly draw on medical/scientific knowledge in their reading of the risk presented, support is normally offered through recourse to anecdotal knowledge ['I had a friend who had the same result']. The potential effect again is to create a community which can offer advice, reassurance – through a variety of genres – and a reading of risk that draws on a creative merging of medical and anecdotal discourses.

While it is fashionable to assert that all texts are polysemic in nature (Fiske 1989) I argue that, while there may be several possible interpretations of a text, the author(s) of any text have in mind a 'preferred' interpretation of what they are saying by their target audience. Looking at what is said by posters in the extracted piece, the discursive strategies that are used contribute to an understanding of 'risk' that may be seen as a *contestation* of expert knowledge. The screening result of 1:2 is negotiated and challenged by others' knowledges and experiences, yet continues to form the backdrop against which questions are formulated and suggestions given. Indeed, when the 'good' result is in, it is seen as a result of 'luck', and not as an expected outcome of a spurious scientific test.

The final section of the discursive analysis continues to look at the meanings generated by textual communication, and attempts to locate the discourse in its broader sociocultural context.

Explanation

This section looks at how the meanings generated in the text contribute ideologically to the perpetuation of power relations (Fairclough 1992; Slembrouck 1998). More specifically, in the context of my research, I will examine how the narrative contributes (or not) to the hegemonic perception of risk found in the medical community. While one must be careful in adducing the 'effect' of a discourse simply from the analyst's interpretation of a text's meanings, there has, nonetheless, been research which suggests that discursive communication – and in particular computer-mediated communication (CMC) – has the potential to transform social relations to the extent that new forms of such relationships might be created (Mason 1989, 1994; Dunlop and Kling 1991). As Kiesler argues, CMC

> brings about qualitative change in how people think about the world, in their social roles and institutions, in the ways they work, and...we say it has transformative effects...because these resources can create educational settings people encounter nowhere else.
>
> (1991: 148)

Indeed, while it is difficult to pinpoint *who* the discourse of risk expressed here may effect (with the web page being a freely accessed public forum), and impossible perhaps to 'separate out' the effect of a text from discursive communication with others in the 'real world', this is not to say that the discussion here does not in itself both reflect and potentially transform/reinforce the ways in which participants calculate the 'risks' associated with screening for 'abnormalities' in pregnancy.

In looking at how discourse analysis seeks to identify the role of discourse in supporting/opposing ideology (Fairclough 1992), it can be suggested that 'expert' knowledges associated with the medical and scientific community might be said to contain ideological elements (Katz-Rothman 1994). For instance, the language of 'risk' in antenatal screening for abnormalities derives not only from existing cultural norms about 'normality', but is shaped and structured by economic and political agendas.[9] There is even evidence to suggest that the backdrop to screening procedures is heavily reliant on NHS cost-cutting, with the cost of caring for a person who has Down's syndrome 'weighed up' against the price of a screening blood test by NHS managers (Wald *et al.* 2003).

If we see such 'expert knowledges' as containing ideological elements, then it is possible to see how the discursive strategies present in the analysed text represent a challenge to the power of the established, hegemonic medical community. The scientifically calculated 'risk' is negotiated and challenged by posters, drawing on a range of strategies: the acquired knowledge of the 'layperson', scientific or otherwise, advice based on professional experience as midwife, and a general need to reassure. Nonetheless, it is striking how, while at one level such strategies work to 'destabilise' the sentiments of the medical expert, the language of risk communicated by posters shares in many ways that of expert discourse. As such it can be suggested that there is some broad agreement as to what the 'risk' to the pregnancy is, the procedures that have to be followed if a definitive result is to be obtained, and a general acceptance of some of the categories that the language of risk reflects and reinforces: notions of 'normality' in both pregnancy, and in the child that is produced, for example.

Indeed, while the strategies in place work at one level to delegitimise the established procedures in place in antenatal screening, it is striking how the risk is resolved only through 'expert opinion' declaring the pregnancy to be normal – a 'false positive'.[10] Indeed, the result is declared to be good luck ('how lucky are we!'), with the flipped coin landing on the 'right' side, and not a predictable effect of what has been considered 'bad science' (Gieryn 1983; see also Note 12). In fact I suggest that what starts as a potentially counter hegemonic challenge to the medicalisation of risk in pregnancy is in the end of little threat to the prevailing medical establishment and its vocabulary of risk. While there are many occasions whereby utterances deconstruct and destabilise hegemonic risk discourses, these fade into the background when the test results are received.

The section which follows develops this theme further, attempting to place my findings into the broader theoretical context of writing on risk society.

Talking through risk: a challenge to modernisation?

Beck has argued that risk should be seen as a systematic way of coping with uncertainty and insecurities created by modernisation itself (Beck and Willms 2004). Evidence for such a statement is twofold from the findings of my research.

First, the development and use of the combined nuchal/blood test for chromosome abnormalities[11] may be seen as a means by which science can be said to rationally cope with the uncertainties and vulnerabilities of nature, with computer programs able to calculate quantitatively the 'risk' of abnormality from a simple blood test. To provide one with a statistical risk might in itself be considered one way of making sense of the unpredictable, with the logical outcome of such classifications extending to the termination of 'abnormal' pregnancies. Risk calculation, for the medical establishment, might thus be considered a way of creating security and control over one's pregnancy, albeit in the broader socio-political context of cultural norms and government agendas.[12]

Second, while the screening test might be seen as a way for science to measure and control nature, in a similar way the communicative discourses considered in my research – what might be considered *perceptions* of risk – might be seen as an attempt to control the insecurities, vulnerabilities and uncertainties *generated through science*. The ways in which the presented 'high risk' is contested and negotiated through the cultural knowledge of the layperson can be seen as a way of coping with the risk calculation generated by the test itself. With security increasingly craved – by both the 'high risk' poster, and those who are supporting her in 'coming to terms' with the risk calculation – we see evidence of Beck's *reflexive modernisation*. Expert opinion and 'science' are, at the very least, put under the spotlight, with the status of scientific knowledge as objective and non-negotiable 'destabilised' through the 'lay-knowledges' and reflexive autobiographies that posters bring to their understanding of risk. Nonetheless, ultimate security is still craved through recourse to science, with Beck's claim that we live in a world in which 'it is impossible not to make decisions, and it is impossible not to make them based on scientific reasoning' (Beck, in Beck and Willms 2004: 54), never ringing so true.

Douglas' work on the role of the institution in shaping the 'thought style' of individuals through the 'classifications' it makes is also useful, and has some relevance in interpreting the behaviour of subjects. Douglas claims that institutions – and we can include in this the scientific community, research firms, governments, the NHS – act collectively to produce knowledge. Such 'knowledge' creates classifications and ways of thinking about the world, which in turn are relied upon by subjects in their decision making. While I would suggest, as Giddens does, that the identities of the posters in my research are by no means established by the certainties that institutions provide (in fact, they are *borne out of vulnerability, insecurity and uncertainty*), the status of the scientific institution as providing both initial 'screening' result, and diagnosis of 'actual' risk, maintains to some extent the reputation of 'science as god', albeit a god that is having to work increasingly hard to sustain its power and legitimacy. To support Beck's thesis, it would appear from my findings that the first and second 'modernities' exist simultaneously, creating an environment in which the need for knowledge of 'risk' and control produces the very insecurities it was meant to prevent.

Reflexive account and conclusions

Just as subjects in late modernity have to 'self-consciously' come to terms with their relation to society, so too must I explore how, as researcher, I relate to my research topic and those involved in communicating 'risk'. In conducting covert *participant* observation, it can be said that I am both subject and object of analysis, contributing through my postings to the text that has been interpreted, while simultaneously stepping 'outside' the discourse in order to discursively analyse that which is being said. As Cresswell suggests, this sort of research approach creates a situation where, epistemologically speaking, 'the researcher and researched are necessarily inseparable and interactive' (1994: 3). While I do not feel that being a researcher who is herself pregnant has shaped my analysis in a detrimental way – with I hope my personal anxieties and worries about risk and pregnancy 'suspended' in the analysis of others' insecurities – this will, undoubtedly, have affected my choice of research topic. Furthermore, I am aware that my experiences and knowledge obtained from my own pregnancies place me in a position that has shaped the questions and answers that emerge in this chapter, and which enable me to 'belong' to the virtual community I study.

A further complicating factor on my identity as researcher has been the covert nature of the research conducted. While initially entering into the discussion forum for research purposes, I have talked, on a day-to-day basis, with the participants and have formed a strong bond through our pregnancies and subsequent early months of life with a young baby. Though I have met several posters from the discussion in 'real life', the research conducted remains covert, a fact that has caused me some degree of guilt and embarrassment. Indeed, it could be suggested that, in researching the vulnerability of others, my own vulnerability as a researcher of risk has come to the forefront: this was felt to be the case in two ways. First, as an academic covertly researching risk in pregnancy, I have found it difficult to remain 'at a distance' from my research subjects. In contributing regularly to group discussions, on all aspects of life, I have in a sense identified more with those that I am studying than with the 'external' role of researcher. As such, to admit now the covert nature of my research would be felt by myself as a betrayal of my role as friend. While being 'found out' is a possible, if remote, outcome, my communication with the group's members is felt to have gone beyond the stage where my research role can be revealed. Second, as pregnant when conducting the research, my own vulnerabilities as a pregnant woman were also heightened when faced myself with the dilemma of antenatal testing. To remind myself of the social construction of risk was of little comfort when faced with my own personal worries and anxieties encountered during this pregnancy.

Nonetheless, despite the ethical issues encountered through the secretive nature of the research practice, it is considered that the benefits of the research vastly outweigh any possible negative effects on research subjects. As has been discussed at length above, in partaking in a publicly accessible discussion forum the information posted is free to be used in any way, without obtaining the consent of those participating in such discussions. Similarly, my own input to the group, which continues to this day, might theoretically be used by another researcher, with an unknown agenda. Or, more fancifully perhaps, my research subjects might too have hidden agendas that have never, and will never, be revealed to myself or to other members of the group!

In terms of the beneficial effects of my research on research subjects, I would argue that in critically exploring the ways in which health care providers present the topic of antenatal testing, and in deconstructing the ways in which risks are manufactured and received, the socially constructed nature of so-called 'scientifically' produced risk might be revealed. In revealing the vulnerabilities of all who are involved in the game of risk, it is possible that those faced with the decision about testing in pregnancy – and indeed those who implement such testing – will be better informed and ultimately empowered through gaining a critical insight into the ways in which – in the words of Beck – uncertainty and vulnerabilities might be considered as *manufactured.*

Notes

1 Economically, it has been calculated that the costs of looking after, for instance, a child with Down's syndrome is vastly in excess of the costs of implementing a screening programme for identifying possible affected pregnancies and, after diagnosis, terminating Down's syndrome pregnancies (Wald *et al.* 2003). Culturally, the drive towards the production of 'perfect' babies, reflected in the immense growth of childcare philosophies and 'how to' guides, conflicts to some extent with the acceptance of a pregnancy that will result in the birth of a child that may have disabilities. Politically, the present government is committed to antenatal screening programmes, having recently encouraged the extension of screening for Down's syndrome for pregnant women of all ages to ensure equity throughout the UK. Former guidelines suggested targeting only women aged 35 plus (ibid.).

2 I reflect later on how Internet chat, perhaps more so than that generated in interviews or focus-groups, is very much reliant on acceptance of that which the poster reveals/conceals. At an extreme level, I had no guarantees that the members posting were themselves actually pregnant, or even female (or they of me). There are interesting parallels here with Baudrillard's notion of the hyperreal (1983), in which subjects exist on the 'surface' of things, underpinned by no objective reality, yet communicating at a level which exists in, even transcends, the 'real' (non-cyber) world.

3 'Singleton' in this context refers to a pregnancy where a single foetus is present.

4 I continue to meet up regularly with fellow-posters, out of personal, as opposed to professional, interest.

5 The 'integrated' or 'combined' test collates the findings of a maternal blood test, looking for 'atypical' markers with the nuchal fold test, an ultrasound scan which measures the thickness of skin-fold at the back of the foetal neck. The combined result can be used to give an indication of the level of 'risk' a woman is at of having a foetus affected by the chromosome 'disorder' Down's syndrome. This 'test' is a screening programme, and the majority of women who have a 'high risk' result will in fact be carrying 'normal' foetuses. An affected pregnancy can only be determined by an invasive test such as amniocentesis or chorionic villus sampling. For a fuller discussion of screening and invasive testing in pregnancy for abnormality, see Katz-Rothman (1994).

6 Such 'control' may itself be mythical, in the sense that we have little say over how what we say or write privately to others might be used and applied.

7 'Moments of crisis', or 'cruces', are considered by Fairclough as a useful point of enquiry, highlighting 'aspects of practice which might normally be naturalised, and therefore difficult to notice; but they also show change in process, the actual ways in which people deal with the problematisation of practices' (1992: 230).

8 Murray (1996) notes that participants in CMC understand the potential for 'flame war' and are often quick to diffuse any possibility that offence might be taken by a statement that is made. Baym (1995), interestingly, suggests that the presence of women is important for the absence of 'flaming' in a group, though my own research across a range of discussion forums does not generally support this claim.

9 The present government requires all hospital trusts to offer screening for Down's syndrome to all pregnant women, regardless of age.

10 The frequency with which 'false positives' arise is rarely discussed or accounted for by the medical establishment.

11 The most common of these is trisomy 21, or Down's syndrome, though the 'abnormal' patterns of bloods the program screens for may read 'high risk' for Patau's and Edwards' syndromes.

12 The accuracy of risk-calculation software has recently been investigated by the National External Quality Assessment System, in partnership with the National Screening Committee project team. The review demonstrated that 'even when consistent results are obtained for biochemical testing, significant differences occur in the risk estimate given to the woman when identical data are fed into the different software packages'. The report concluded that 'The feasibility of offering a personalised risk estimate will be explored' (National Screening Committee 2003: 14).

References

Baudrillard, J. (1983) *Simulations.* New York: Semiotext(e).

Baym, N.K. (1995) 'The emergence of community in computer-mediated communication', in S.G. Jones (ed.) *Cybersociety: Computer-mediated Communication and Community.* Thousand Oaks, CA: Sage.

Baym, N.K. (1998) 'The emergence of online community', in S.G. Jones (ed.) *Cybersociety 2.0.* Thousand Oaks, CA: Sage.

Beck, U. (1992) *Risk Society: Towards a New Modernity.* London: Sage.

Beck, U., Giddens, A. and Lash, S. (1994) *Reflexive Modernisation: Politics, Tradition and Aesthetics in the Modern Social Order.* Cambridge: Polity.

Beck, U. and Willms, J. (2004) *Conversations with Ulrich Beck.* Cambridge: Polity.

Bordia, P. (1996) 'Studying verbal interaction on the Internet: The case of rumour transmission research', *Behaviour Research Methods, Instruments and Computers* 28(2): 149–51.

Cresswell, J. (1994) *Research Design: Qualitative and Quantitative Approaches.* Thousand Oaks, CA: Sage.

Douglas, M. (1986) *How Institutions Think.* Syracuse: Syracuse University Press.

Dunlop, C. and Kling, R. (1991) 'Social relationships in electronic communities', in C. Dunlop and R. Kling (eds) *Computerization and Controversy: Value Conflicts and Social Choices.* Boston: Academic Press Inc.

Fairclough, N. (1992) *Discourse and Social Change.* Cambridge: Polity.

Fiske, J. (1989) *Reading the Popular.* London: Routledge.

Giddens, A. (1990) *The Consequences of Modernity.* Cambridge: Polity.

Gieryn, T. (1983) 'Boundary-work and the demarcation of science from non-science: Strains and interests in professional ideologies of scientists', *American Sociological Review* 48: 781–95.

Grinyer, A. (2002) 'The anonymity of research participants: Assumptions, ethics and practicalities', *Social Research Update* 36: 3.

Herrera, C. (1999) 'Two arguments for "covert methods" in social research', *British Journal of Sociology* 5(2): 331–43.

Hewson, C., Yule, P., Laurent, D. and Vogel, C. (2003) *Internet Research Methods: A Practical Guide for the Social and Behavioural Sciences.* London: Sage.

Homan, R. (1991) *The Ethics of Social Research.* London: Longman.

Howard, T. (1993) 'The property issue in e-mail research', *Bulletin of the Association of Business Communications* 56(2): 40–1.

Jones, S.G. (1995) 'Understanding community in the information age', in S.G. Jones (ed.) *Cybersociety: Computer-Mediated Communication and Community.* Thousand Oaks, CA: Sage.

Katz-Rothman, B. (1994) *The Tentative Pregnancy: Amniocentesis and the Sexual Politics of Motherhood.* New York: Rivers Oram Press.

Kiesler, S. (1991) 'Talking, teaching, and learning in network groups: Lessons from research', in A.R. Kaye (ed.) *Collaborative Learning through Computer Conferencing: The Najaden Papers.* Springer-Verlag/NATO Scientific Affairs Division, Berlin.

Mason, R.D. (1989) 'A Case Study of the Use of Computer Conferencing at the OU'. Unpublished PhD thesis.

Mason, R.D. (1994) *Using Communication Media in Open and Flexible Learning.* London: Kogan Page Ltd/Institute of Educational Technology.

Murray, P.J. (1996) 'Nursing the Internet: A Case Study of Nurses' Use of Computer-Mediated Communications'. MSc Dissertation.

National Screening Committee (2003) *Antenatal Screening for Down's Syndrome – Policy & Quality Issues.* Available at http://www.screening.nhs.uk/downs/dssp_policy.pdf.

Norris, J. (1994) 'The way we were at 31 Oct', *NURSENET* – A Global Forum for discussion of nursing issues [online], LISTSERV@VM.UTCC.UTORONTO, CA.

Slembrouck, S. (1998) *Multi-media and the Internet – A Project for Discourse Analysis.* Available at http://bank.rug.ac.be/da/mmda.htm

Wald, N.J., Rodeck, C., Hackshaw, A.K., Walters, J., Chitty, L. and Mackinson, A.M. (2003) 'First and second trimester antenatal screening for Down's syndrome: The results of the Serum, Urine and Ultrasound Screening Study (SURUSS), *Health Technology Assessment* 7(11): 2.

Chapter 8

Constructing virtual selves

Men, risk and the rehearsal of sexual identities and scripts in cyber chatrooms

Anthony Pryce

This chapter is concerned with same-sex, erotic, 'online' activities of men who use Internet sex chatrooms but who may not yet, if ever, define themselves as gay or even bisexual. These erotic activities often breach the borders of hegemonic masculinities and may involve the individual in a reconstruction of social identities and sexual performativity, especially for a man who had considered himself to be heterosexual or 'straight'. The apparent dissonance of men who identify as straight and married, but who have sex with men, is not a new phenomenon (Kinsey *et al*. 1948; Humphreys 1970), nor is it uncommon (Pathela *et al*. 2006). With the Internet now ubiquitous as a freely available means of transmitting and consuming erotic imagery and engaging in sexual interaction, the opportunities for same-sex activity have expanded, yet the organisation of chatroom sexualities remains potentially risky, requiring practical organisation and discretion management that require them to learn new forms of interaction.

Although, at least superficially, virtual sex may mirror some aspects of a *real-world* physical encounter, it appears largely free of the personal and social vulnerability, physiological constraints or health risks associated with embodied erotic interaction. However, the individual actor may graduate to engaging new forms of desire and practices into both their online and offline sexual activities, and they are increasingly vulnerable to numerous potential threats that demand some (re)construction of their calculations of health and social risks as well as their sexual identity.

For those men who are, or have become, 'curious' about sex with other men, online activities can render the individual actor vulnerable in a number of ways. A study by Pathela *et al*. (2006) of straight-identifying men in New York revealed that 12 per cent of married men had same-sex encounters in the previous year, and suggested that men whose sexual identity is discordant with their sexual behaviour may engage in riskier sexual behaviours than those with concordant identity and behaviour (Kelly *et al*. 2002). Bisexual men, it is suggested, could play an important role in the spread of sexually transmitted diseases, not least because they constitute a hidden population and less likely than gay men to have relevant knowledge about AIDS and safer sex. However, Weatherburn *et al*. (1998) found that behaviourally bisexual men often did have quite good knowledge of HIV risk.

However, because they appear not to share a common notion of sexual identity, let alone community, they are not identifiable as a group, thereby hard to target in safer sex campaigns. This concern with the 'risk' posed by bisexual activity accents the deep scepticisms generally expressed in both gay and straight populations with the problematic nature of the bisexual identity itself, where 'Bisexuals [are] depicted as "fence sitters" who were in essence homosexual and who distanced themselves from this identity to benefit from "heterosexual privilege" and to avoid stigmatization' (Weinberg *et al.* 1994, in Weinberg *et al.* 2001: 183). Clearly such ambiguities and tensions at the heart of bisexual identity and practices are central to discourses about the 'fixed' versus constructionist notions of (bi)sexuality. I am also assuming here that sexual identities, or at least sexual behaviours, are more fluid or contextual than the essentialist binary categories suggest. However, the emotional and psychological implications resulting from the cybersexual challenge to lifelong assumptions about the 'fixed' or 'natural' basis of their sexual desires and orientation might have far reaching consequences. It exposes the individual to risks that are located in the Internet interaction itself. There are social risks that might ensue from problematising his familiar interior sexual and emotional geography, and which may provoke radical reconstructions of the sense of self, identity and practices in everyday life offline. Social risks include the destabilising of previous emotional and sexual relationships such as marriage or a potential loss of employment if the actor is discovered engaging in inappropriate sex chat online at work. A most obvious risk is acquiring sexually acquired infections through offline 'meets'. Not least in these risk discourses is the construction of new pathologies of 'cyber addiction' that also serve to reinforce existing moral anxieties around sexual consumption, deviance and fidelity. This dense mesh of risk requires even the most naïve of users to learn a new set of scripts to manage both the online interactions and their offline consequences.

Much of the focus in this chapter draws on a recent qualitative, ethnographic study that has provided rich evidence of the online and offline experience of some men who identify as heterosexual, bisexual or 'curious' and often also married or partnered. It focuses on how they use Internet chatrooms, apparently as a means of exploring and testing out their erotic desires and fantasies. Central to the mapping of the virtual encounter is what this might mean in terms of the calculation and management of the multiple risk factors involved in Internet sex chatrooms as new performative spaces to rehearse and explore other sexual identities. It is useful to provide a brief overview of some methodological concerns and theoretical influences that provide valuable opportunities for reading this densely interwoven matrix of themes and substantive issues. However, the main thrust of this discussion concerns how Internet-based sexual activities have been variously constructed as 'risky', especially as a threat to the heteronormative social order as evidenced by the vociferous online sites that draw on religious, moral and other medico-psycho-social discourses that pathologise forms on transgressive Internet use. I will focus rather more on the data analysis from *real-time* electronic interviews. These explore ways in which these men learned and developed their use of the chatroom and the management of their social roles within the public/private sexual arena. I will outline a description of sexual career trajectories of chatroom users and also suggest how these processes emerge and are nuanced in response to the risks that permeate these potentially stigmatising and transgressive erotic practices.

In conclusion, I propose that this analysis of empirical data suggests men use Internet sex chatrooms for a number of purposes. One key factor may be the opportunity that the easy access provides for the instrumental examination of the actor's own sexual identities and desires with the co-presence of other actors, supposedly within a relatively safe anonymous social setting. This may be true, but such voyeuristic activities and self-surveillance may result in more than simply being the passive consumer of sexual imagery, where pictures and text fuel erotic activities and fantasies that can signify significant shifts (or resistances) in the pursuit of desire. Rather, it is a socially constructed arena, a computer-mediated[1] rehearsal space, dense with agency where the actor learns scripts, rules, behaviours and identities that the participant may then relocate in embodied offline performances.

Constructing the problem of risk and cybersex

Particularly through the 1990s the Internet, particularly the ease of availability of porn and sex-based chatrooms, was rapidly identified as the locus for emotional, social and sexual risks, spawning a considerable industry predicated on the pathologising and medicalising consequences of cybersex use. 'APB', an online tabloid that focuses on crime, headlined an article 'Fleeting Thrills or Cybersex Addiction?'. It argued that a large percentage of obsessive-use patterns have a sexual component such as porn sites, sex-related chatrooms and cybersex. Edelson (2000) also suggests there are 300,000 adult sites, cybersex sites and sex chatrooms online. Among the themes that the article sought to explore was 'whether sexual compulsion online leads to sex crimes offline?', thereby reiterating the putative association between the dark power of cyberspace to influence, adversely, individual agency in the 'realworld'. One example from the rise of such discourses in the late 1990s illustrates the tendency to pathologise the cybersexual.

Questions and Answers:
Sex and Lust Department
Please remember, this column is designed to help the consumer seeking behavioral-health information, and not intended to be any form of psychotherapy or a replacement for professional, individualized services. Opinions expressed in the column are those of the columnist and do not represent the position of other SHPM staff.

Question
My husband is addicted to on-line cybersex. This has been an ongoing problem for many months now. Can you help?

Answer

Sadly, this is becoming a more common problem every year. As with most compulsive behaviors, addiction to on-line cybersex is often a response to anxiety that is an attempt to avoid or escape personal problems, social distress or unpleasant emotions. It involves a sense of shame because of an inability to control the compulsive behavior, in this case, a preoccupation with and strong desire for sex that involves downloading sexually explicit material, spending hours in sex chatrooms, bulletin boards, etc. to the extent that occupational and social spheres are disrupted.

Self Help Magazine 03/18/98 (http://shpm.com/qa/qasex/qasexcyber.html)

Clearly, for many people the realisation that their partner spends many hours in highly sexualised activities, albeit mediated through virtual interaction, represents a significant stressor and risk to the relationship. In response, a significant online array of psychological/counselling services, virtual clinics and therapies have foregrounded cyberaffairs and the increasing risks associated with ease of access to sex sites and porn and cybersex addiction. Lupton (1999: 35) identifies this 'major threat to moral and social order' as a realist epistemological position. Tracking the popularity and accessibility of the Internet, articles increasingly appeared on *Net*.porn, such as that in *Men's Health* magazine (July/August 2000), which outlined the risks to jobs, relationships and the technology itself through viral contagion. Paradoxically, the article then provided addresses of 'top ten porn sites' including schoolgirls4u.com and porncity.com before going on to demonstrate how to eliminate traces so that employers and partners cannot detect the transgression!

Cybersex is pathologised, constructed as an addiction that can be treated within the same paradigmatic approach as Alcoholic Anonymous (AA) and other self-help, confessional recovery regimes to become 'Web Sober'.[2] The dominant heteronormative assumptions are evident in the concern with infidelity and the discursive formation of sexual desire being coterminous with social role and identity. However, little or no regard is given to behaviours or desires of the actor for whom online interaction may be part of a socially transformative process as well as a mode of self-fashioning or self-actualising of the self suggested by Foucault's (1979) 'ethical subjectivity'. In the erotic diasporas of the chatrooms, these participants may not just be adulterous. They may also be exploring virtual desires, and perhaps through 'meets' (organised 'real' encounters) physically engage in erotic practices that do not just challenge conventional models of adultery in heterosexual marriage, but also transgress and destabilise what may have been hitherto a rigidly defined sexual orientation and identity in the 'real' world.

There are, of course, resistances to the dominant discourse on individual websites.[3] However, the reproduction of offline forms of both sexual consumption and economy has not adequately problematised the liminal, 'the transitional, middle stage between two distinctly different entities or sites' (Lupton 1999: 133). This is particularly relevant in relation to bisexuality, which as Storr (1999) demonstrates as both theory and social identity in postmodernity is problematic, unstable and contested as a social state. On the one hand, the actor engaged in online sexual activities is concerned with *Ars Erotica* (Foucault 1979), the processes around which the individual actor may be concerned about the truths of his own experience and sometimes the formation of a transgressive sexual identity. *Ars Erotica* encompasses the activities, careers and imaginations of the individual and their erotic biographies and performativity. Conversely, the apparatus of the online 'Netaddiction.com' culture represents the deployment of technologies and governmentality of the *Scientia Sexualis* (Foucault 1979). Such liminal individuals or collectives such as immigrants, refugees, bisexuals or gays transgress and threaten conventional boundaries. On the net, as in the real world, they become objects of hate, disgust or fear (Ling 1996).

There is no doubt that, together with the consumption of porn as text and image, the participation in a spectrum of cybersexual erotic encounters is extensive and also lucrative. Whilst mindful of the critics of the potential of sexual and social dangers of the chatrooms, Thompson (2000) argues that large domestic Internet Service Providers (ISPs) such as AOL and Compuserve require and facilitate this sexual economy. There is, however, evidence to refute the notion that users of chatrooms are dysfunctional isolates (Hamman 1997), that they seek replacements for offline community by joining communities online. Gutfield (2000) cites one study of 9000 people (of which 85% were male) who used 'adult' websites; about half spent less than one hour a week online for sexual purposes. A substantial literature of cyber sociology has begun to emerge that maps the construction of the Internet and the production and reproduction of porn (Harmon and Boeringer 1997), the social structures of chatroom communication (Donath *et al.* 1999), and user nicknames and aliases (Bechar-Israeli 1995). Other studies have included Foucauldian analyses of Internet discourse (Aycock 1995), narratives of experiencing cyberaffairs ('Sue', 1997), relationship and friendship development (Parks and Floyd 1996), the conduct of cyber ethnographies (Paccagnella 1997; Dicks and Mason 1998), humour in chatroom interaction (Bechar-Israeli 1995) and ethnographies of gay sex chatrooms (Shaw 1997). A particularly helpful study of predominantly heterosexual cybersex chatroom sites was conducted by Hamman (1997), computer-mediated telling of interactive sexual stories (in real time) with the intent of arousal.

The access to new sites of sexual potential clearly raises a number of questions. For example, to what extent does Internet chat provide a basis for testing out sexual fantasies as a tentative step towards transition from solitary fantasy to 'real' embodied shared interaction? One risk is the dangers of technological infection by viruses in a supposedly safer zone stemming from increasing consumption of diverse sexual practices, notably the transfer of porn images carries with it the greatest risk of computer viruses! To what extent is the online sexual environment with its potential for ongoing refinement and rehearsal of sexual personae consistent with Foucault's notion of the *Ars Erotica*? In terms of orientation for many men the focus and agency of their online sexual desire is entirely consistent with their offline biographies, sexual histories, fantasies and practices. As Shaw (1997: 133) suggests in his study of gay men and computer communication, the texts produced by the actors online is, 'like Barthes's love, discourses of absence'. In the Goffmanian sense, the self is a reflexive constitution by and of the social world. Thus the cyber-self, no less than its embodied counterpart, may be argued to be produced through ritual, through the practices and relations which constitute the intersubjective fabric of the online social world. If an actor tries to influence the perception of his image, this activity is called self-presentation. This of course has attendant risks that render the individual potentially vulnerable to 'leaking' information such as revealing phone numbers or other personal details from their 'real' offline world to the online community. Surprisingly, given the perception of *weirdos* and dangerous individuals stalking the Net, individuals are often quite trusting. The conventional notion of the individual acting within social frames would appear to be problematic in the online context of community. How valid is the notion of continuities between the online and offline communities (Watson 1997)? While Mitra's study was of an Indian online community there is some room for translating this into the way sex participants mediate their offline community with the online diaspora. Once familiarised with the social world though, it seems that people feel safe in sexually explicit online environments (Witmer 1997). Nevertheless, beginning as married/partnered men with a heterosexual identity in the offline world, how do they learn the complex strategic activities that may lead to new identities as 'bicurious', 'bisexual' or 'gay', and their development of the instrumental management of multiple risks?

Risky (cyber)bodies and virtual identities

A fundamental question is whether the use of chatrooms is merely a cyber-playground for a voyeuristic consumption of sexual stimulation and erotic curiosity, or does the chatroom become a means of meeting others and make the leap from cybererotica to *realworld* sex? Is this a means of confirming sexual orientation (e.g. as 'really' being or becoming heterosexual/gay/bi/'open-minded' etc.) through developing social networks and acquiring the skills for the management of discreditable and potentially dangerous identities, both physically and socially? It can be argued that, for some men seeking sex with men, danger is a contributory *erotic charge* in cruising (Rechy 1963, 1967, 1977; Bech 1997), whereas to some extent the organisation on the Net of meetings for sex reduces some of the risk and *frisson* of the sexual hunt. A paradox remains at the heart of the process however, which is that, whilst the process of exploring sexual desire through Internet-based interactions might be 'empowering' for the individual, it is clear that the act(s) of *becoming a cybersexual* is suffused in risks to individual and social safety in terms of physical, sexual and mental health. I want to give emphasis here to the actors' *virtual* sexual careers and (loosely) following Benner (1984) the movement from *bi-curious* 'novice to expert' sexual actor. This provides the basis for a reconsideration of what constitutes 'risk' in virtual encounters and the development of tentative categories of social identities and cyber-cultural sexual practices. There are many echoes here with Goffman's theories on the management of self and social interactions (1959, 1963, 1967) and also the ethnographies of public sex from the 1960s and 1970s (Pryce 1996).

People do not usually behave as if free to undergo significant changes such as taking on different sexual practices, orientation or identity, without reference to the performance of their expected social roles, especially where any such deviation might violate powerful social constraints. Thus, an important feature of the research concerned men's discretion management of online sexual experiences and embodied activities and explored how social and sexual health risk is constructed, calculated and managed in relation to the tensions of their offline–online social roles and sexual identities. Some men seemed happy to present themselves using the commonly recognised chatroom category of 'openminded' to suggest a kind of erotic agnosticism or, perhaps more sceptically, sexual opportunism. Analyses suggested that despite 'everyday' world social categories and a priori sexual identities as 'heterosexual', 'married' or 'bisexual', men utilise chatrooms for a variety of purposes (Tikkanen and Ross 2003). For some men, this may become strategic in terms of reconstructing less prescribed sexual scripts, practices and identities whilst acquiring new forms of social knowledge and perhaps even intrapsychic insight (Simon 1996; Simon and Gagnon 1999). For example, a key set of elements that influence both the conduct and construction of online performance and offline social 'realities' are the various strategies employed by the actor to lessen or avoid the potential risks associated with this pursuit of desire(s).

The study by Weinberg et al. (2001: 183) identified a number of problems when considering taking on and maintaining a bisexual self-identity which seemed to follow stage-like processes:

> notably, gays and lesbians were said to reach an endpoint in which their sexual preference identity became relatively clear and permanent. Bisexuals in our research did not show such closure. In particular, negative social reactions and questions about the whole notion of bisexuality from other sexual communities fueled recurring feelings of uncertainty, with no apparent closure with respect to the identity. For example, gays and lesbians questioned whether bisexuality and a bisexual identity had the potential to persist.

As I go on to explore here, there are resonances with the findings in the study where, although stages of transition may be readily identified both behaviourally and socially, there are persistent questions about both the essentialist and constructionist readings of sexual desire, praxes and identity. In the panoptic spaces of both the contemporary home and the Internet, the pursuit of erotic desire and 'authentic' self is in discursive tension with the controlling of dangerous sexualities through technologies of governance. On the one hand, there has been the increased incitement to engage with the project of *askësis* (the pursuit of individual sexual truth and pleasure) and the use of technologies of the self in *Ars Erotica* (Foucault 1979: 57) in the construction of identity. On the other is a parallel, associated discourse that implicates the strategic use of the Internet as a means of organising sexual encounters with the increased risk of disease, such as syphilis (Bull and McFarlane 2000; CDC 2003; Taylor *et al.* 2005).

Researching the *re*-materialisation of sex

Sexualities and erotic practices are 'succumbing to digital dematerialisation' (Walby 1998), and this study draws on the increasing literature on cyber research, particularly ethnographies of public sex. The research explored three key questions:

1   How do married/partnered men learn to use Internet sex chatrooms when the content/object of desire involves transgressing offline sexual identities?
2   Does the cyber environment become a new performative rehearsal space for sexual activities, fantasies, practices and identities that subsequently may be enacted in *real* life offline?
3   What are the techniques and modes of governmentality that operate at the *risky* interface of two discursive formations, offline identity and cyber realities?

In attempting to undertake enquiry into social practices that are produced through the mediation of computer technologies, the methods used need to be appropriate and embedded in the naturally occurring data. In this case, it is the chatroom that is the *foreign* territory for the ethnographic gaze. Numerous practical guides are now available that assist the virtual ethnographer, given the differences between researching online environments from *real* world settings (Hamman 1997; Dicks and Mason 1998; Cavanagh 1999; Mann and Stewart 2000). As Coomber (1997) argues, there may be significant research benefits for developing new knowledge where the group being researched is normally difficult to reach, and/or the issues researched are of a particularly sensitive nature. This is especially so when the respondents may neither accept nor relate to offline definitions or identities such as 'bisexual' or 'gay'. Chatroom users, when online, can adopt a variety of assumed biographies and identities, such as a gay man who may adopt 'str8 married' status, which for some men may heighten their desirability as a potential sexual partner. However, as Hamman (1996) notes, the process of undertaking research on actors who may transform themselves into multiple characters is problematic. Similarly, Turkle argued that 'virtual reality poses new methodological challenges for the researcher; what to make of online interviews and indeed whether and how to use them' (1995: 324). The reliability of narrative accounts of sexual activities or the constructions of online–offline continuities is not an issue in this study. Rather, the research is more concerned with the men's use of the rooms as performative social spaces and their narratives of engagement with other men. Thus, whilst the text is central here to the capturing of the online scripting of cybersexual life, I would echo Plummer's (1995: 16) concern that the narrative story telling is 'socially produced in social contexts by embodied concrete people experiencing the thoughts and feelings of everyday life'.

The research was conducted in two phases. First, the 'covert' non-participant phase was undertaken, exploring the territory, describing the ecology and getting familiar with the argot, the social rules and patterns of behaviour. Covert observation in ethnographic research has been increasingly regarded as ethically questionable over the last few decades where some studies, such as Humphreys' study *Tearoom Trade* (1970) about sex in public toilets, produced spectacular results but would not obtain ethics approval nowadays! The central argument against covert methods is that it invades privacy, there is no opportunity for the 'subject' to give informed consent and there may be a danger of breach in confidentiality or anonymity. In terms of Internet research there are further echoes of the ethnographies of the 1960s and 1970s, where 'exotic' deviant subcultures were observed and documented with little problematisation of methodological and ethical considerations. Thus, as the Internet emerged in the 1990s as a popular and accessible new medium and consequently spawning increasing academic interest, the pioneering literature on digital cultures initially paid scant interest to ethics, although that is now rapidly changing in response to the explosion of interest in both the methodological opportunities of the Internet as well as substantive research subject(s) (Shields 1996; Hewson *et al.* 2003).

A pivotal issue for all ethnographies lies in how the public/private boundaries are nuanced in ethical research. As early ethnographies of sexual spaces demonstrated, the term 'public' is contested (Pryce 1996), but here it carries two main interpretations:

1   Spaces in the social domain that are potentially accessible to actors who, by virtue of their apparent role(s), may claim to have a legitimate presence in that space; and
2   Those elements of observable performance in which are encoded rules, meanings and regulatory behaviours that mediate (potential) sexually laden action.

Such public spaces, particularly those centred on illicit and transgressive behaviours, require the neophyte participant to gain an understanding of the rules. It is no different for researchers when entering the cyber field, and Berry (2004) identifies what this means in terms of ethical conduct. He does effectively argue for flexibility and illustrates the frequent role of (non-researcher) 'lurkers' on sites to which they subscribe but do not contribute. Similarly, when exploring the ethical and methodological concerns in 'netnography', and drawing on communications studies and market research, Beckman and Langer (2005) effectively articulate the fundamental issues. They summarise these key tensions in 'netnography', which is 'based primarily on the observation of textual discourse', but where the divisions between public/private discourses are far from clear. They go on to argue that from an ethnographic perspective covert research might be an appropriate methodology, in particular when studying sensitive research topics. Similarly, Lee (1993: 143) takes a pragmatic view, recognising potential difficulties associated with covert research. It acknowledges the need to protect the rights of research participants and the obligation not to harm them, but still accepts covert studies, in particular if there is no other way for the necessary data to be obtained.

In the case of this study, covert observation was seen to have some value in revealing hidden or unknown aspects of social interaction and agency, and therefore a pragmatic position was taken. The decision to include a period of covert observation in this study of online groups and interaction was based on two key aims. First, a period of adjustment or 'decompression' (Delph 1978) is helpful for the researcher, just as when the individual in daily life takes a while to make sense of the scene when entering any new and potentially unfamiliar environment. Second, the traditional argument that Berry (2004) cites, that the 'subjects' being observed might change their behaviour if they knew, does make sense and was therefore regarded as a robust basis for having a short phase of covert observation whilst also rigorously guarding the participants' anonymity.

During the initial exploratory phase, three main chat services, mIRC (Internet Relay Chat), Microsoft Chat and 'gaydar.co.uk', were considered suitable research sites. At the start of the study, Microsoft Chat was the one most likely to be used by new or inexperienced Internet users ('newbies'), as it was factory-loaded onto new computers for the domestic market, but has now been suspended as a chat service in the UK. Gaydar.co.uk is another one that is commonly used by married men, partly as it is also easy to access and traces of its usage can be discreetly controlled. mIRC is another channel that can be accessed by free downloading (for more confident users) or could have been discovered via Microsoft Chat. However, experience suggested that the most fruitful site that attracted the widest range of users was gaydar.co.uk, and a fourth, much smaller gay/bisexual chatroom site, chrisgeary.co.uk, appeared to attract a number of men who identified as married or curious. During the descriptive and exploratory phase, the nickname 'curious' was employed to engage in conversation with other participants but excluded cybersex activities. To some extent, many of the difficulties associated with offline ethnographic practice apply here, such as the dangers of *going native* but also maintaining ethical boundaries.

Phase two involved the direct recruitment of 70 men over the age of 17, who demonstrated a good use of spoken English, for real-time online interviews. They were given information electronically about the project together with how their confidentiality and other ethical implications of research will be ensured. They were asked to 'sign' an online consent form that stipulates that the research will not involve engaging in cybersex. There is of course no certain way of checking the veracity of the interview narratives; however, the issue is less on the verifiable 'truth' but rather how these men told their stories.

Only twelve men wished to be interviewed by phone, the rest involved online, real-time computer-mediated communication (CMC). The participants' ages ranged from 17 to 63 years, of which the majority were aged between 24 and 43 years. Of those who stated their ethnicity, three were black Afro-Caribbean, five were south Asian, Indian and Bangladeshi, and seven were of Asian origin that included men of Thai, Malaysian and Taiwanese origin living in the UK. There appeared to be a broad spectrum of social class with occupations, when disclosed, that included plumbers and construction workers, military and other service personnel, university academics, graphic designers, computer technicians and computer software designers, doctors, students, salesmen and also a number of unemployed. Out of the total number interviewed, 46 were married, 13 lived with or were involved with long-term relationships with girlfriends, seven were divorced or separated whilst the remaining four were living at home with parents and, of these, two denied having had offline sexual experiences with either women or men. All the participants stated that they used chatrooms on a regular basis, often involving the exchange of porn images, erotic chat leading to masturbation through text-based cybersex, and 'fonewank' or camera-to-camera-based (C2C) erotic display that usually leads to ejaculation. Some used the chatrooms as a way of either routinely, or occasionally, finding partners for offline sex.

In terms of sexual orientation, only four identified as 'bisexuals' who were 'out' to their female partners; 31 admitted to adolescent same-sex experiences involving masturbation; and 48 stated that, as adults, they had some erotic offline encounters with men either as a result of chatroom talk/cybersex or other non-Internet meetings. Many of these men described how they had tried to curb both homoerotic fantasies and sexual encounters with men once they were married. However, for some men there had been either strong desires to extend their sexual repertoire with new experiences, which most suggested were happening now because such activity or desire had hitherto been 'suppressed', or as a result of 'changes' in sexual interests. A few expressed same sex or other specific erotic interests that they had not acted on previously but 'thought about' for many years, whilst a minority of men seemed to manage a complex 'double life' of casual sex. Those encounters could be arranged online or achieved through 'cottaging' (picking up men in public toilets), cruising known sex venues such as parks or simply as a result of serendipitous encounters in hotels whilst working away from home. Through the interviews it emerged that, in terms of fitting these men into any kind of notional categories, 12 men could be identified as bi-curious, 25 as gay and the remaining 33 constitute bisexuals.

The ethnography of digital sex

Many of the married men interviewed saw the acquisition of an Internet-ready computer as an increasingly necessary and useful household tool, especially for their children. However, it was also an opportunity to explore aspects of their sexuality that had hitherto remained erotic arenas within solitary masturbation activities or memories of earlier desired or actual experiences. For those who are not particularly technically skilled, most modern home computer kit is Internet-ready and requires little skill to gain access to the Web. The computers are loaded with the more family-targeted Internet Service Providers (ISPs) such as AOL, but these usually include chat groups that are easily accessible such as Microsoft Chat or gay.com with a wide diversity of interests. For those not familiar with the practices of online sex chatrooms, it appears on the one hand to be a potential sweetshop of erotic consumption. On the other, it is a wild frontier where external laws are invalidated but where there remain rules of conduct and interaction to be learned.

Gaydar.co.uk is easily found and accessed if the actor is searching for same-sex chat and it provides a portal to both the virtual and offline gay social, sexual and economic 'community', having many links to other gay sites and is itself also widely advertised offline. There are numerous channels organised around global geographical locations. The UK and Ireland channel was used in this research, and it contains rooms by country, city and area, as well as a list of rooms of 'specialised' interest. These include 'Bears', 'Bisexual', 'Bondage', 'Buddhists', 'Christians', 'Couples', 'Curious', 'Cyber', 'Deaf Men', 'Fantasy', 'Locker-room', 'Married Men', 'Masseurs and their Clients', 'Military', 'Muscle', 'Music and Arts', 'Muslims', 'Phone', 'Soccer Players and Fans', 'Sports Kit', 'Straight Men' and 'Suits and Ties' as well as particular sexualised uniformed groups such as 'Gay Cops' or 'Air Crew' and also categories for couples (of unspecified genders), escorts and commercial sex workers.

To some extent the self-identification of practices, preferences, intentionality and desires are displayed in the nicknames that are adopted and these may change through the rehearsal, repetition and refining of identity(ies). Indeed the nickname may be a statement of intentionality or destination but not yet have been enacted offline, nor indeed online, but is an accommodation of a potentially new sexual identity. Examples of user profiles or brief self-descriptions include:

- Lee, b'mouth, virgin pvt: im married in brighton
- Norfolk guy; 45 new to this so looking for a guy to help me. I love oral but want more
- Simon 40 Devon: married bi-guy seeks discrete fun/friendship

The nicknames may also make statements not just of orientation but also specific fetishes; physical boundaries; whether they can travel; who phones whom; whether they can provide or need accommodation; geographical location; timing; whether it is essentially a commercial transaction; or a potential emotional as well as sexual encounter. The self-statements usually carry some textual representation as physical type of self or preferred other. When opening chatroom interactions, the most common mode of initial interaction is 'a/s/l?' (age/sex/location), which is followed by a more elaborate description focusing on sex characteristics. On Gaydar.co.uk the initial interaction tends to be more discursive, picking up a comment based on the actor's self-profile or some other greeting such as 'how u doing?'. Age is significant and for some men it is an organising element, such as for those only desiring younger or older; for some, maturity is problematic and the actor may try and pass as much younger than he is. Evidence from the research suggested that many of the men who are beginning to significantly question or address their 'core' sexuality tend to be over 30. In some chatrooms attempts to obtain pictures or interact with much younger men (teen or preteen boys) are monitored and users banned if they transgress. Other rooms are clearly facilitating adult men's interest in younger males and vice versa.

Chatroom performance involves numerous, sometimes fragmented, coded processes. Not least is the actor's ability to 'multitask' by writing text responses in conversation with maybe two or more people concurrently. These texts include the development and presentation of what is often a frequently rehearsed, constructed biography, that over time and with the acquisition of performative skills may be highly edited and interwoven with elements that emphasise some form of sexual attraction. The central motif of the chatrooms is the erotic and the eroticising of the interaction engagement. Generally the scripting revolves around being 'horny' and banter that is intended to move quite quickly on to disclosing particular sexual interests, fantasies, recounting real life sexual experiences, the individual's current state of arousal including descriptions of his body, particularly focusing on genitalia and what is the intention of the other's presence: is it for chat, cybersex, phone sex or to arrange a meet? This process may also include the transmission of 'self-pics' that may or may not be authentic pictures of the actor who may simply be sending on pictures that he received from somebody else and is now *passing* as himself. Such interactions may take a few moments when abbreviated to:

A: hi...a/s/l
B: [replies]
A: horny? CALL ME...[tel number]

Mobile phones tend to be most readily used as a more expensive, but safer, option than giving out domestic landline numbers. This may extend to men who use the chatrooms from work, engaging in cybersex from their desk and use the office phone to call out. It seems that many men in offices, and also home-workers, are almost constantly online in chatrooms, monitoring them whilst also engaged in legitimate work. When I have asked people's occupations some were often employed as computer technicians and software programmers, but the range of employment by men who were online at work included engineers, architects, local authority workers, accountants, solicitors, dentists, doctors, academics and retail workers. In this respect there is a tendency for men in higher social class work to have privacy and access to Internet time that may usually be unmonitored. Men who usually only logged on from home did so during the day if they were working from home, on a day off, night/shift workers, on holiday or when the wife/partner was away at work. Class stereotypes and characteristics also sometimes featured in nicknames and sex preferences with references to 'blue collar' or occupations associated with physical labour and implied 'rough' sexiness such as work associated with a uniform. Paradoxically, it seems that many men who used their own home computers more for chatroom use tended to be in lower paid/status jobs and therefore they spent more on Internet use. The peak time for chatroom use was lunchtime, when some men came home for lunch or some used Internet cafés to try and arrange immediate or early evening 'meets' before going home. Other peak times are early evening and late night; frequently the interactions occur when partners and/or children are asleep.

There were other variations in the social constituency of users. In US-based chatrooms, colour and ethnicity appear much more central, indeed almost the organising element, in defining both the identity of the chatroom user and their preferred 'other'. However, in the UK white users rarely mentioned their colour but other ethnic and racial groups did. Afro-Caribbean men seemed to be far less visible than Asian or Indian men and these were all far outnumbered by men who were assumed to be white.

A fundamental question remains, 'What is available and how does cybersex occur?' As I suggested earlier, I would argue that Hamman's definition of cybersex can be extended to articulate more nuanced practices that may be helpful in chronicling chatrooms as performative and rehearsal spaces. More specifically the process of becoming a cybersexual may involve a number of 'developmental' stages that can be identified by the ease or willingness with which men might utilise the various computer, telephone or face-to-face interactions. The most common repertoire of cybersex activities may be represented as:

- text-based curiosity and tentative enquiries
- text-based interactive story telling, erotic arousal and masturbation
- cybersex
- phone sex
- microphone/computer-mediated text as one-2-one or 'public'
- camera-to-camera (C2C)
- meeting offline for drink or friendship or maybe sex
- meeting specifically for offline sex.

For some men there are clear preferences for how and when each one or more may be enacted. For some men their use of text-based interaction or phone might signify a linear progression that both reflects and drives their changing career trajectories. In many cases it would seem that they are expedient much more on immediate, practical circumstances. These primary methods may be enhanced through the use of conference facilities such as Yahoo Messenger or MSN Messenger, both of which help the actors by enabling rapid e-mail, one-2-one chat and the transfer of files, such as photographs. Video interaction is increasingly accessible using digital cameras that are now routinely bundled with new computers. These messengers also provide 'friends' lists whereby a network of contacts can be maintained and which also alert the cyber user when another friend is online or logs on. The analyses of the data suggested that there is a close relationship between willingness to engage in cybersex performance, and in the ways in which men construct and adopt sexual identities.

Cybersexual praxes, identities and career trajectories

Three main arenas of praxis, the Novice, Experimenter and Expert, were identified and provide a useful means of charting the net.sex users' career, in what I have described as a pedagogy of the cybersexual. The cybersexual categories for the purpose of the focus on men who use the chatrooms for same-sex activities include the 'bi-curious', 'bisexual' and 'gay'. Unsurprisingly the Web use of 'open-minded' as a legitimate identity and orientation presents a slight problem because of its ambiguity and ambivalence. In practice, as well as simply being a less contentious identity than 'bisexual' (Storr 1999), it seemed from the data that the concept was adopted primarily by men who had sex with men but for whom the hint of appearing predominantly straight would enhance their potential attractiveness to others. For the purposes of this chapter I have, for convenience, regarded 'open-minded' as bisexual.

It might appear that the cybersexual careers that I am describing here are somewhat reductive with some linear drive or progression, implying that categories are fixed, determined and stable. However, they are remarkably dynamic as within these basic organising categories a number of significant social roles are played out at the capillary level with a range of scripts, rules and modes of performativity. Clearly, the question may be asked where divisions in categories are transformative; for instance, at what point does the bi-curious expert become an experimenting bisexual? In addition, the performative exposure to other more elaborated practices may influence the actor so that their progression is not linear and uni-directional but may move categories. Indeed, some men revealed how they observed their own cycles of engagement and would have periods of quite intense activity and then retreat or 'take fright', subsequently to return a few months later and restart the cycle. The issue here, however, is the construction of risk and discretion management that is demanded in the conduct of each of these trajectory moments.

Bi-curious (n=12)

The chatroom novice may be a 'newbie' to both Internet use and same-sex desire and activities; sometimes their interest has been stimulated through watching porn and even for the first time observing another man's erection. The user tends to be tentative, looking for commonalities with others, and whilst expressing desires and fantasies may have little or no offline experience. These men may have spent considerable time searching for, and using, porn sites as a consumer before venturing into chatrooms, initially as a 'lurker' (non-participant observer).

As an experimenter he gains familiarity with online argot and the 'netiquette' required to navigate the new erotic territory within which he may develop 'strong' online relationships that include cybersex. He may engage in phone sex but many of the narratives in the study suggested that they preferred a narrow range of erotic scenarios to be shared with the other person. This often includes exploring bisexual scenarios such as MMF (two men and a female) as the organising theme for erotic chat. For some men, that provided a relatively 'safe' stabilising and legitimate motif to engage with other men, whereas for others, the primary concern was with the other man. At least in fantasy, some men talked of including their female partners or wife in three-way activities, or a desire to watch another man have sex with her. However, it seems this was rarely disclosed and less often acted on and most men usually remained secretive, risk averse and cautious in the disclosure of information. However, many enjoyed being a voyeur of others who are willing to 'show' on cameras.

The expert may go on to use cameras in two-way interaction (C2C) and might arrange an offline 'meet'. Whilst men may accept a shift or altered sense of self-identify, many of the bi-curious men appear to retain a 'straight' sexual role that remains largely within heteronormative hegemonic male power relations. Most of the men in this group suggested that their primary interest in same-sex activity was genitally focused, with several claiming that they did not actively 'fancy' other men. All the men said they enjoy watching or participating in a range of sexual practices such as masturbation, and a few even anal sex, but generally as the 'active' partner, although some experimented with and enjoyed a 'passive' role. However, most were adamant that they were not looking for emotional, romantic involvement and did not want to kiss other men. Whilst all confirmed that, if revealed, their activities would be deeply stigmatising. However, almost unanimously they rejected suggestions that their offline identity and masculinity was compromised by 'just wanking' with other men and that they often preferred to be with men of the same social class and with similar interests. Indeed, the majority of these men admitted to preferring the idea of casual sex with 'other married blokes' because of the reduced risk of exposure as each party 'knows the score'. Indeed, a few of the men in the bi-curious group expressed confidence in their ability to arrange or construct sexual encounters with men offline, although opportunistic encounters were reported where alcohol often acted as a disinhibiting factor.

Bisexual (n=33)

Many of the novice bisexual men interviewed reported having had previous offline experiences, often before their marriage or living with their partner. Although a large number admitted to sometimes or predominantly using homo-erotic masturbatory imagery, many had not acknowledged same-sex interest until accessing the Internet. This group widely reported self-awareness of having 'other' desires yet subject to a strong sense of social/sexual controls on both the desire and its practice. Younger men seem to regard bisexual experience as emancipatory and more legitimate than the older men who tended to identify with essentialising sexual categories of greater, more pronounced polarity. Of these older men, several felt that they were beginning to accept a change in their identity and that they were allowing their 'real' feelings and behaviours to emerge.

The experimental bisexual men tended to routinely use both gay and straight porn, and swap 'self pix' (sometimes facial but usually body and genital pictures). Most of the men reported how, in their early phase of active discovery of other erotic practices, they extended their repertoire of sexual imagery, ideas and fantasies. They increasingly engaged in cybersex and developed new interests for practices such as oral sex, with occasional or frequent use of phone sex, but many wished to move on to the 'real thing'. To this end, many men reported having sought some initiation with a 'safe' tutor. Especially for men in remote or non-metropolitan areas, many used chatrooms to contact others and several discussed having one or more regular sex partners as well as 'one-off' chance encounters. Most of these men (who were not 'out' bisexuals) maintained their marriage but required subterfuge to conduct both their cyber and offline sexuality as in any adulterous encounter.

The expert bisexual men utilised the chatrooms as a resource for organising and planning immediate and future sexual activity. Whilst these men reported a broadening of their access to other bisexual/gay resources and increased the purposeful use of chatrooms, many said that their forms of interaction had become more restricted to camera use once chatroom contact had been made. Clearly for them, there was now a fluency with chatroom culture, roles and expectations and they regarded them as a relatively easy way to arrange and manage 'meets'. They reduced the risks associated with 'cruising' or 'cottaging' or other potentially discrediting activities, especially in rural or non-gay areas. However, when visiting on business and for the men in larger towns and cities, many bisexual men used commercial gay bars, saunas and other 'cruising' environments. Several of these men did identify as 'bi', having come out to their female partner, and a few claimed that their female partners were occasionally or routinely involved in threesomes. Four of the men interviewed claimed that their partners had played a part in their change of sexual interests as a result of their wife's initiation of sexual experimentation, which had resulted in the husband being able to explore sexual activities with the second man whilst within the 'safety' of the 'acceptable' triangle. However, some men did manage their marriage relationship without disclosing and the risk of 'discovery' was a commonly given reason why many of the men preferred sex with other married men who would 'know the score'. For many of the men the wife's work pattern or periods of separation provided a framework to organise sex opportunities. Many of the bisexual men did express a desire to seek an emotional 'relationship', while a third of the interviewees described one or more long-term or 'sex-buddy' relationships, some of which involved romantic attachments.

Gay (n=25)

The novice gays were usually younger men, or older men who claimed that they were now discovering their 'real' self. Many were, or had been, married with several admitting that they had suppressed their sexual desires and activities at marriage for the sake of their partner, to be 'normal' and to avoid the risk of stigma. Several men had identified as 'bisexual' when young, partly because it had been more acceptable, even fashionable, as a sexual lifestyle choice and left the options open as a way of avoiding difficult labels, such as 'gay'. These men all admitted to becoming increasingly aware of new or revisited same-sex interests and desires, and for some this had taken place over a number of years. Nearly all these men have had some previous same sex experiences such as a single encounter with a 'straight' best friend at school or university that had created a deep and lingering erotic and/or emotional resonance over time. At least half the men had moved quite rapidly from a tentative, bi-curious (re)entry point through to bisexual experimenting and now verging on taking a gay identity. Throughout that process most had sought to understand the commercial and social gay ecology, places such as bars/saunas. Those who were married had not necessarily disclosed their shift in sexual practices to their partner and fearing loss of access to children and other significant life changes continued to conduct sexual encounters covertly. The progression to being gay experimenters seemed to continue seamlessly for many of these men. They used chatrooms for cybersex, phone sex and meets and many had 'usernames' signifying explicit sexual interests or desires that often represented a refining of erotic interests. For the majority of these men, gay sex was now the primary interest; although several maintained their marriage, some admitted that there had been a significant reduction in sex with their wife often over a long period before chatroom activities began. However, half the men had disclosed their new sexual identity to their wife, often suggesting that this is part of gaining a more 'authentic' self.

As an expert the *rites de passage* into a gay identity with knowledge of much of the commercial gay ecology has been experienced, sometimes by men who even a few months earlier might have never admitted to same-sex erotic fantasies or activities. The chatrooms are now central to the access and structure of that ecology as a means of providing a sex-'organiser' for meets or cyber or phone sex. The Internet user has become familiar with other sites online and the local gay scene offline and their social network is more likely to include gay friends. Most of these men identify as 'out' gay and have disclosed their orientation to their wives, some of whom appear to be willing to tolerate the change either for the sake of continuity in the family and/or because of emotional attachment. However, 12 of the men reported that they were now separated or divorced since disclosure.

Conclusions

Learning how to tell a sexual story and to test or rehearse a 'borrowed' identity whilst gaining an understanding of the social ecology of the Internet is to engage in a pedagogy of the cybersexual. In other words, those 'straight' men who start using Internet porn and chatrooms, and then begin to explore their own sexual boundaries, need to learn (with the direct or indirect participation of others) how such desires and practices can be conducted within the role expectations of both the Internet communities and offline society. These forms of conduct to some degree reproduce offline rules; maybe a desire for order on the frontier land works to construct a simulacrum of socially defined modes of interaction and the impression of stability in the presentation of self. The notion of simulacra is particularly appropriate when exploring the *virtual* world of the Internet and, in this case, the destabilising of lifelong, gendered and sexual performativity. Drawing on the concept developed by Baudrillard, the simulacrum of everyday life is evident where society has replaced all reality and meaning with symbols and signs, and that in fact all that we know as 'real' is actually a simulation of reality. In 'postmodern' cultures the appearance of reality provides endless opportunities for both intended and unintentional manipulation of the surface of things – plastic looks like wood, a hotel in Las Vegas appears to be Venice, and the movie *Matrix* is based on elusive and mutable notions of 'reality'.

Similarly, the pedagogical progress of the cybersexual also facilitates the construction and maintenance of disguise stories and strategies for degrees of revealing or disclosure. Part of the strategies discussed by participants in the study echo early ethnographic research of illicit or 'deviant' sexual identities and practice. These are the transitions between everyday activities and the 'other', or what Delph (1978: 9) called the 'decompression zones' as the boundaries, spaces or processes or time frame that allow the passage of the individual from the site of discrediting activity to the *outside* world. A key point here is the extent to which sex chatrooms have become public performative spaces.

The data suggests there are a number of purposes for cyber use including the project of *askësis* or the sexual career of the individual actor. It is a social space with specific and contextual modes of interaction, with complex scripts and inter/textualities. There are a number of clear processes of biographical (re)construction and narrative forms within chatrooms. In the case of the men in this study, their sexual direction and online identities are not stable but constructed through the process of learning to be (cyber)sexual. However, as Weinberg *et al.* (2001) found in their study of bisexuals at mid-life, contrary to popular belief, the bisexual identity can be stable and people who self-define as bisexual are not necessarily 'in transition' towards another sexual preference identity.

Even so, there is evidence that the Internet chatrooms are used to test out, explore, reveal and refine ideas, and explore new potential and behaviours that may or may not be translated into the offline setting. Most contentiously, of course, it could be argued that such careers are deeply destabilising, they erode heteronormative assumptions and foreground the contested notion of bisexuality and the fluidity of sexual desire. It is apparent that these findings require more work to effectively theorise a number of important themes.

First, it is important to explore further how the various practices and risks identified here engage with new modes of governmentality. For example, how does the presentation of the actor reproduce moral paradoxes of the public/private where cybersex is a threat to the dominant offline order? Associated with this are a number of questions that stem from the role of the body in the cybersexual encounter. How is the body variously conducted and reconstructed to comply with fantasies and forms of narrative? How also does resistance to these often troubling, sexualising tensions operate? Certainly, resistance is found in the frequent 'toe in the water' behaviours of many of these men at each 'stage' of the career where a point of erotic saturation is reached or where the lure of the 'other' is rejected when it threatens the everyday framework of the family, social status or other familiar signifier of well-being.

Second, from the perspective of sociologists of health, it is valuable to explore the discursive practices of medicine in defining the pathological and deviant around Internet-based erotic agency. Here the calculation of health risks, for example the construction of net.*addiction* and the conceptual reconstruction of invisible populations *at risk*, requires signficiant consideration. At the heart of this concern lie further questions about the normative aspects of cybersexual activity that may, paradoxically, be obscured by the emphasis on the exotic and deviant. The cyberworld is both real and transitory; it has no time, yet is bound by temporal mechanisms and boundaries of its individual users. It is essentially a social and, as I have argued, a public space that is available for the rehearsal and performance of multiple encounters and the (re)construction of biographical narratives through the production of computer-based texts and the calculation of multiple layers of risk. Clearly, the actions and performativity of the cybersexual online may have a significant impact on the agency of the actor offline. It is particularly in this complex interchange of powerful, and often competing, desires and forms of social control that governmentality in the form of *risk* is both deployed and resisted.

Notes

1   This is not a 'techie' chapter and, to some extent, the technology is irrelevant except for what and how it enables the actor to pursue in terms of increasing possibilities for individual and social changes, interactions and opportunities for rehearsing hidden, suppressed, transgressive or stigmatising sexual/emotional practices. Use of terms like online and offline as *argot* conveniently and economically differentiate between interactions in chatrooms, e-mail or other computer-generated media such as MSN Messenger, and those offline interactions such as telephone and physical meetings. To some extent, this avoids epistemological problems such as the notion of 'real' interaction as opposed to 'cyber'.

2 The Center for On-Line Addiction produced a brochure, 'Getting Web Sober: Help for Cybersex Addicts and Their Loved Ones' (http://www.netaddiction.com).
They outline the content of the brochure that can only be sold online:

When Fantasy Turns into Obsession

- How to evaluate addiction using the Cybersexual Addiction Index (CAI) – a 20-item assessment tool
- How to deal with recovery when Relapse is a Mouse Click Away
- How to Practice Healthy Internet Use Management
- How to Evaluate Server and Software-Based Solutions
- Signs of Healthy Cybersex Use
- How Families can intervene to break a loved one's denial with a seven step plan.

3 See for example a gay site that refutes such definitions of addiction and its negative effects: http://www.gaymenscounselling.com/cybersex2.html

Bibliography

Aycock, C. (1995) 'Technologies of the self: Foucault and Internet discourse', *Journal of Computer Mediated Communication* 1(2). Available at http://jcmc.indiana.edu/vol1/issue2/aycock.html (accessed June 2007).

Bech, H. (1997) (trans. T. Mesquit and T. Davies) *When Men Meet: Homosexuality and Modernity*. Cambridge: Polity.

Bechar-Israeli, H. (1995) 'From <Bonehead> to <Clonehead>: Nicknames, play, and identity on Internet relay chat', *Journal of Computer Mediated Communication* 1(2). Available at http://jcmc.indiana.edu/vol1/issue2/bechar.html (accessed June 2007).

Beckman, S. and Langer, R. (2005) '*Netnography*: Rich insights from online research'. Available at http://frontpage.cbs.dk/insights/pdf/670005_beckmann_langer_full_version.pdf (accessed June 2007).

Benner, P. (1984) *From Novice to Expert*. Menlo Park: Addison Wesley.

Berry, D. (2004) 'Internet research: Privacy, ethics and alienation. An open source approach', *Internet Research* 14(4): 323–32. Available at http://opensource.mit.edu/papers/berry2.pdf (accessed June 2007).

Blythe, M. and Jones, M. (2004) 'Human computer (sexual) interactions', *Interactions* 11(5): 75–6.

Bull, S.S. and McFarlane, M. (2000) 'Soliciting sex on the Internet: What are the risks for sexually transmitted diseases and HIV?', *Sexually Transmitted Diseases* 27: 545–50.

Cavanagh, A. (1999) 'Behaviour in public? Ethics in online ethnography', *Cybersociology* 6. Available at http://www.cybersociology.com/files/6_2_ethicsinonlineethnog.html (accessed June 2007).

CDC (2003) 'Internet use and early syphilis infection among men who have sex with men, San Francisco, California, 1999–2003', *MMWR* 52: 1229–32.

Coomber, R. (1997) 'Using the Internet for survey research', *Sociological Research Online* 2(2). Available at http://www.socresonline.org.uk/2/2/2.html (accessed June 2007).

Delph, E.W. (1978) *The Silent Community*. London: Sage.

Dicks, B. and Mason, B. (1998) 'Hypermedia and ethnography: Reflections on the construction of a research approach', *Sociological Research Online* 3(3). Available at http://www.socresonline.org.uk/3/3/3.html (accessed June 2007).

Donath, J., Karahalios, K. and Viégas, F. (1999) 'Visualizing conversation', *Journal of Computer Mediated Communication* 4(4). Available at http://jcmc.indiana.edu/vol4/issue4/donath.html (accessed June 2007).

Edelson, E. (2000) 'Fleeting thrills or cybersex addiction? Experts warn of a new affliction', in C. Hurlburt and M. Wallace (1999) 'Pornography on the Internet: The Red-Light District of Cyberspace', *Concerned Women for America*. Available at http://www.cwfa.org/printerfriendly.asp?id=2001&department=cwa&categoryid=pornography (accessed June 2007).

Elford, J., Bolding, G. and Sherr, L. (2001) 'Seeking sex on the Internet and sexual risk behaviour among gay men using London gyms', *AIDS* 15(11): 1409–15.

Foucault, M. (1979) *The History of Sexuality, Vol.1*. London: Penguin.

Foucault, M. (1989) *Foucault Live (Interviews 1966–84)*. New York: Semiotext, Columbia University.

Gates, B. (1996) *The Road Ahead*. New York: Viking.

Goffman, E. (1959) *The Presentation of Self in Everyday Life*. New York: Doubleday.

Goffman, E. (1963) *Behaviour in Public Places: Notes on the Social Organization of Gatherings*. New York: Free Press/Macmillan.

Goffman, E. (1967) *Interaction Ritual*. New York: Pantheon.

Goffman, E. (1974) *Frame Analysis: An Essay on the Organization of Experience*. New York: Harper and Row.

Gordon, C. (1991) 'Governmental rationality: An introduction', in G. Burchell, C. Gordon and P. Miller (eds) *The Foucault Effect: Studies in Governmentality*. Chicago: University of Chicago Press, pp. 1–52.

Gutfield, G. (2000) 'Welcome to porn.com', *Men's Health* 6(6) (July/August): 92–7.

Hamman, R. (1996) 'Cyborgasms: Cybersex Amongst Multiple-Selves and Cyborgs in the Narrow-Bandwidth Space of America Online Chat Rooms'. MSc Thesis, University of Essex. Online at http://www.cybersociology.com/files/cyborgasms.html (accessed June 2007).

Hamman, R. (1997) 'The application of ethnographic methodology in the study of cybersex', in *Cybersociology*, 1(1). Available at http://www.cybersociology.com/files/1_1_hamman.html (accessed June 2007).

Harmon, D. and Boeringer, S. (1997) 'A content analysis of internet-accessible written pornographic depictions', *Electronic Journal of Sociology* 3(1). Available at http://www.sociology.org/archive.html (accessed June 2007).

Haubrich, D.J., Myers, T., Calzavara, L., Ryder, K. and Medved, W. (2004) 'Gay and bisexual men's experiences of bathhouse culture and sex: "Looking for love in all the wrong places"', *Culture, Health and Sexuality* 6(1): 19–29.

Hewson, D.C., Yule, P., Laurent, D. and Vogal, C. (2003) *Internet Research Methods*. London: Sage.

Humphreys, L. (1970) *Tearoom Trade*. London: Duckworth.

Jones, Q. (1997) 'Virtual-communities, virtual settlements and cyber-archaeology: A theoretical outline', *Journal of Computer Mediated Communication* 3(3). Available at http://jcmc.indiana.edu/vol3/issue3/jones.html (accessed June 2007).

Kelly, J.A., Amirkhanian, Y.A., Mcauliffe, T.L., Granskaya, J.V., Borodkina, O.I., Dyatlov, R.V. *et al.* (2002) 'HIV risk characteristics and prevention needs in a community sample of bisexual men in St. Petersburg, Russia', *AIDS CARE* 14(1): 63–76.

Kinsey, A.C., Pomeroy, W.B. and Martin, C.E. (1948) *Sexual Behavior in the Human Male*. Philadelphia: W.B. Saunders.

Lee, R.M. (1993) *Doing Research on Sensitive Topics*. London: Sage.

Ling, R. (1996) 'Cyber McCarthyism: Witch hunts in the living room', *Electronic Journal of Sociology* 2(1). Available at http://www.sociology.org/content/vol002.001/ling.html? PHPSESSID=9b02b09332786 (accessed June 2007).

Lupton, D. (1999) *Risk*. London: Routledge.

Mann, C. and Stewart, F. (2000) *Internet Communication and Qualitative Research: A Handbook for Researching Online*. London: Sage.

Mitra, A. (1996) 'Nations and the Internet: The case of a national newsgroup, "soc.cult.indian"', *Convergence: The Journal of Research into New Media Technologies* 2(1): 44–75.

Mitra, A. (1997) 'Diasporic web sites: Ingroup and outgroup discourse', *Critical Studies in Mass Communication* 14: 158–81.

Mitra, A. (1999) 'Characteristics of the WWW text: Tracing discursive strategies', *Journal of Computer Mediated Communication* 5: 1.

Paccagnella, L. (1997) 'Getting the seat of your pants dirty: Strategies for ethnographic research on virtual communities', in *Journal of Computer Mediated Communication* 3(1): 267–88. Available at http://jcmc.indiana.edu/vol3/issue1/paccagnella.html (accessed June 2007).

Parks, M.R. and Floyd, K. (1996) 'Making friends in cyberspace', *Journal of Computer Mediated Communication* 1(4). Available at http://jcmc.indiana.edu/vol1/issue4/ parks.html (accessed June 2007).

Pathela, P., Hajat, A., Schillinger, J., Blank, S., Sell, R. and Mostashari, F. (2006) 'Discordance between sexual behavior and self-reported sexual identity: A population-based survey of New York City men', 19 September, *Annals of Internal Medicine* 145(6): 416–25.

Plummer, K. (1995) *Telling Sexual Stories*. London: Routledge.

Pryce, A. (1996) 'Researching Eros – revisiting ethnographic chronicles of male sex in public places', *Sexual and Marital Therapy* 11(3): 321–34.

Rechy, J. (1963) *City of Night*. New York: Grove Press.

Rechy, J. (1967) *Numbers*. New York: Grove Press.

Rechy, J. (1977) *The Sexual Outlaw*. London: Futura.

Sannicolas, N. (1997) 'Erving Goffman, dramaturgy, and on-line relationships', *Cybersociology* 1. Available at http://www.cybersociology.com/files/1_2_ sannicolas.html (accessed June 2007).

Shaw, D.F. (1997) 'Gay men and computer communication: A discourse of sex and identity in cyberspace', in S.G. Jones (ed.) *Virtual Culture: Identity and Communication in Cybersociety*, pp. 133–145. London: Sage.

Shields, R. (ed.) (1996) *Cultures of Internet*. London: Sage.

Simon, W. (1996) *Postmodern Sexualities*. London: Routledge.

Simon, W. and Gagnon, J.H. (1999) 'Sexual scripts', in R. Parker and P. Aggleton (eds) *Culture, Society and Sexuality*. London: UCL Press, pp. 29–38.

Smith, C.B. (1997a) 'Conduct control on Usenet', *Journal of Computer Mediated Communication* 2(4). Available at http://jcmc.indiana.edu/vol2/issue4/smith.html (accessed June 2007).

Smith, C.B. (1997b) 'Casting the Net: surveying an Internet population', *Journal of Computer Mediated Communication* 3(1). Available at http://jcmc.indiana.edu/vol3/issue1/smith.html (accessed June 2007).

Storr, M. (1999) 'Postmodern bisexuality', *Sexualities* 2(3): 309–25.

'Sue' (1997) 'New to cyber liaisons', *Cybersociology* 1. Available at http://www.cybersociology.com/files/1_4_sue.html (accessed June 2007).

Taylor, M., Montoya, J.A., Cantrell, R., Mitchell, S.J., Williams, M., Jordahl, L. *et al.* (2005) 'Interventions in the commercial sex industry during the rise in syphilis rates among men who have sex with men (MSM)', *Sexually Transmitted Diseases* 32(10), supplement: S53–S59.

Thompson, N. (2000) 'Sex in the digital city: Why it's so alluring on AOL and the Internet – why it's so addictive', in *The Washington Monthly Online.* Available at http://www.washingtonmonthly.com/features/2000/0007.thompson (accessed June 2007).

Tikkanen, R. and Ross, M.W. (2003) 'Technological tearoom trade: Characteristics of Swedish men visiting gay internet chat rooms', *Aids Education and Prevention* 15(2): 122–32.

Turkle, S. (1995) *Life on the Screen: Identity in the Age of the Internet.* New York, NY: Simon and Schuster.

Waites, M. (2005) 'The fixity of sexual identities in the public sphere: Biomedical knowledge, liberalism and the heterosexual/homosexual binary in late modernity', *Sexualities* 8(5): 539–69.

Walby, C. (1998) 'Circuits of desire: Internet erotics and the problem of bodily location', in R. Diprose, R. Ferrell, L. Secomb and C. Vasseleu (eds) *The Politics of Erotics.* New York: Routledge.

Watson, N. (1997) 'Why we argue about virtual community: A case study of the phish.net fan community', in S.G. Jones (ed.) *Virtual Culture: Identity and Communication in Cybersociety*, pp. 102–132. London: Sage.

Weatherburn, P., Hickson, F., Reid, D.S., Davies, P.M. and Crosier, A. (1998) 'Sexual HIV risk behaviour among men who have sex with both men and women', *AIDS Care* 10(4): 463–71.

Webb, S. (1999) 'Cyberspace as everyday life', in *Cybersociology* 6 [currently offline].

Weinberg, M.S., Williams, C.J. and Pryor, D.W. (1994) *Dual Attraction: Understanding Bisexuality.* New York: Oxford University Press.

Weinberg, M.S., Williams, C.J. and Pryor, D.W. (2001) 'Bisexuals at midlife: Commitment, salience, and identity', *Journal of Contemporary Ethnography* 30(2): 180–208.

Witmer, D.F. (1997) 'Risky business: Why people feel safe in sexually explicit on-line communication', *Journal of Computer Mediated Communication* 2(4). Available at http://jcmc.indiana.edu/vol2/issue4/witmer2.html (accessed June 2007).

Chapter 9

Reframing risk

How risk discourses are used by Vaccine Critical groups in the UK

Pru Hobson-West

This book covers a wide range of topics but all are linked to the themes of health, risk and vulnerability. The focus of this chapter is vaccination, and more specifically organized parental resistance to mass childhood vaccination in the UK. Drawing on empirical data, the main aim of the chapter is to investigate how risk is constructed by 'Vaccine Critical groups' (Hobson-West 2005). I argue that risk is constructed in several ways and that these combine to challenge the dominant vaccination discourse. Before proceeding, some introductory points are necessary in order to clarify how the topic relates to the broader themes of the book.

In terms of *health*, vaccination is credited with achieving dramatic reductions in morbidity and mortality from infectious disease. For the public health profession, vaccination is regarded as 'a cornerstone of preventive medicine' (Streefland 2001: 159) and the eradication of smallpox is celebrated as 'one of the greatest public health success stories' (Poland and Jacobson 2001: 2440). Vaccination is also considered to be a very cost-effective public health intervention (Ehreth 2003). *Mass* vaccination requires high population uptake in order to promote 'herd immunity', defined as a situation where disease circulation is blocked, thus protecting all in the community, including those who are not fully immune (McGuire 1998). In this way, the actions of individuals are said to have potential health benefits for the wider population. Vaccination in the UK is organized by the state, led by the Department of Health, and administered and supported by the medical profession.

Vaccination is also closely linked to the topic of *risk*. If understood simply as hazard, then risk is relevant in that vaccine technology is an attempt to reduce the incidence of one particular type of hazard: that is, disease. More interesting, however, is the way that comparative risk is used as a strategy to encourage public compliance with the national recommended schedule (Department of Health 2004). This use of risk is commonplace in health promotion campaigns. In the case of vaccination, the risks associated with vaccines are presented as lower than the risks from exposure to disease (Hobson-West 2003). Compliance with vaccination programmes is thus constructed as the rational decision. Those who oppose vaccination are assumed to have misunderstood this fundamental equation (Bedford and Elliman 1998). Opposition to vaccination has also been explained as resulting from an individualist approach to risk (Rayner 2002; Hodge and Gostin 2003) and a failure to appreciate the community benefits of vaccination compliance, as promised by the concept of herd immunity.

Social scientific exploration of vaccination has increased in the last few years, partially in response to significant declines in uptake of the measles, mumps and rubella (MMR) vaccine and intense media debate in the UK. This controversy is often blamed on the publication of a paper by Wakefield and colleagues of the Royal Free Hospital in London. The paper, published in the high profile *Lancet* journal, was a preliminary report of a clinical study which suggested that there may be a link between MMR, a type of autism and bowel disease (Wakefield *et al.* 1998). In response, the government continue to recommend the combined MMR vaccine and maintain that 'the overwhelming weight of evidence proves that MMR is safe, and the number of studies demonstrating this is growing' (NHS 2004). The methods of Wakefield's paper have been attacked as 'clinical anecdote' and Wakefield himself has also been accused of a conflict of interest related to aspects of his research funding (Deer 2004). Dr Wakefield resigned from his post in 2001 but stated that 'I have been asked to go because my research results are unpopular' (BBC News 2004).

The MMR controversy has arguably increased the general level of public concern around childhood vaccination. A procedure that for some parents may have been a relatively routine part of child-rearing has now become a topic to agonize over and a moment of potential danger. Recent empirical research confirms that parents do express fear and anxiety, and worry about making the right decision for their child (Brownlie and Howson 2005; Poltorak *et al.* 2005). This results in a situation where 'MMR talk' has become a social phenomenon in itself (Poltorak *et al.* 2005). More specifically, the anxiety induced by vaccination could be analysed in terms of *vulnerability*, the third theme of the book. In short, although childhood vaccination is designed to protect the vulnerable from threats or risks to health, one could argue that vaccination itself is now associated with feelings of vulnerability.

From a broader theoretical perspective, this reported anxiety about MMR could be analysed as just one of many anxieties that characterize life in contemporary risk society (Beck 1992; Wilkinson 2001). The risk society thesis also includes the idea that science itself will increasingly become recognized as the source of risks that we are now struggling to manage. This appears to apply to the MMR case and the feared risk of autism. According to the risk society theory, traditional norms no longer hold. One consequence is further anxiety and vulnerability, as 'the individual increasingly stands alone, looking for security in the face of uncertainty and an implosion of knowledge-systems' (Annandale 1998: 19). Some of these important theoretical issues will be returned to at the end of the chapter.

Before moving on it should be stressed that, whilst the MMR controversy and media debate form part of the context of this research project, they are not the focus of the discussion here (see Hargreaves *et al.* 2003; Harrabin *et al.* 2003).

The chapter does not claim to investigate public, parental or 'lay' attitudes (see Poltorak *et al.* 2005; Brownlie and Howson 2005, 2006). Rather, what follows is based on an empirical study of organized groups who campaign against aspects of childhood vaccination in the UK. Contemporary groups of this sort have not been subject to much detailed analysis, but are discussed elsewhere in relation to trust, and existing published accounts of historical vaccination opposition (Hobson-West 2007).

Of the three themes – health, risk and vulnerability – what follows is primarily focused on the second of these. The chapter adopts a social constructionist approach by investigating whether and how discourses of risk are used. The findings suggest that risk is an important theme for the Vaccine Critical groups, but only in the sense that they are engaged in challenging and reframing the dominant risk discourse. In other words, the reframing of risk is part of the political strategy of the groups. This reframing is achieved in five different ways: by stressing unknowns; questioning the relationship between individual and community risk; constructing risk as manipulated; challenging the benefits of vaccination; and focusing on further vaccine-related conditions. After reviewing the literature on competing approaches to the study of risk and detailing the research methodology, the chapter presents the data that relate to each of these critical discourses.

Approaches to risk

The literature which discusses risk and health is vast and it is therefore helpful to distinguish between realist and constructionist approaches, with the recognition that this dichotomy is inevitably an over-simplification. Realist understandings of risk are dominant in scientific and technical domains such as epidemiology and in 'cognitive science' approaches such as psychology (Lupton 1999). The risk or probability of a harmful event is calculated and compared with the risk and benefits of another course of action. In the realist view, risk communication refers to the last stage in the process, and follows the identification of a hazard, assessment of risk, and risk management. In response to the communication of expert risk information, the rational risk-minimising individual is expected to adapt their behaviour.

The recognition that the public do not always respond 'rationally' has led to increasingly complex attempts at explaining the apparent difference between actual, objective risk, and risk perception. For example, research in the so-called psychometric tradition (Bennett 1999: 6) has identified 'media triggers' and 'fright factors' (see also Spier 2001) which claim to explain why risk perception is amplified in certain circumstances (Pidgeon *et al.* 2003). Bauer summarizes this approach critically: 'empirical risks (objective risks) are compared with perceived risks and deviations between the two are diagnosed as deficits in non-expert reasoning' (Bauer 1995: 396).

Broadly speaking, social constructionist approaches stress the social and cultural context of risk assessment, and also the constructed nature of risk itself. The contention is that risk is not an objective fact that is out there and waiting to be measured by science. Rather, 'what we measure, identify and manage as risks are always constituted via pre-existing knowledges and discourses' (Lupton 1999: 29). The implication is that expert risk judgements are socially constructed, just as lay ones are, and that all knowledge, even scientific or medical knowledge, is always partial or incomplete. To draw a distinction between real risk and risk perception therefore misses the point. For researchers using a social constructionist approach, the key research question is less about what factors (cognitive, behavioural, emotional etc.) influence risk perceptions, and more about what types of claims are used to construct particular ideas of risk and about the social and political consequences of these claims.

Research that is part of this tradition includes work that focuses on the idea of uncertainty or unknowns. In the realist approach, uncertainty and unknowns may well be recognized but are normally framed as temporary phases that are overcome by more (scientific) research. In contrast, Wynne (1992), amongst others, has argued for distinctions to be made between risk and uncertainty, ignorance and indeterminacy. What this analysis implies is that public concern about a technology, or non-compliance with risk advice, may not be due to a misperception or misunderstanding of that risk, but instead may represent a response to inherent uncertainty or ignorance that has not been taken into account in the statistical calculation. Some empirical evidence exists for this in relation to genetically modified (GM) food. According to Marris and colleagues it is precisely the denial of inherent uncertainties, especially about long-term or chronic impacts of GM, that accounts for some of the public mistrust of the technology (Marris *et al.* 2001: 87).

Another implication of taking a social constructionist perspective is that risk loses its automatic association with objectivity and neutrality. For example, a critical governmentality approach is powerful in its capacity for reinterpreting risk as political. Far from an objective or neutral result of scientific inquiry, risk assessment facilitates 'government at a distance' (Petersen and Lupton 1996: 19). In short, risk allows health promotion activities not to be seen as direct intervention, coercion or punishment by the state. Instead, risk is a tool that encourages individuals to practise self-regulation (Brown 2000). In the vaccination case, a governmentality approach would highlight how risk is used to encourage public compliance, without the need for direct state sanction. In short, power is still relevant but is more implicit (see Dew 1999). This chapter does not adopt a governmentality perspective but does utilize a broad constructivist approach. In particular it proceeds from the assumption that risk statistics are the result of social processes, and are not simply a technical matter. Examples of resistance to risk advice should therefore be studied as a critical questioning of these processes, rather than as examples of technical misunderstandings.

Methodology

Through a combination of literature review, website searches and snowball sampling, ten organized parental groups were identified in the UK (see Hobson-West 2005). These groups fit two main sampling criteria: first, the groups chosen hold a 'critical' view of vaccines or some aspect of childhood vaccination policy; second, they consider vaccination to be a key topic of concern. Vaccination resistance is therefore relatively narrowly defined. This allows for a more in-depth analysis and is considered justified, given the current lack of existing published research on organized resistance.

The groups are geographically spread and were established at different times, some dating back to the 1970s. The groups are: Action Against Autism (AAA); Allergy induced Autism (AiA); Association of Parents of Vaccine Damaged Children; Informed Parent; Justice Awareness and Basic Support (JABS); Justice for All Vaccine Damaged Children (JFAVDC); vaccination.co.uk; Vaccination Information; Vaccine Awareness Network (VAN; now called Vaccine Information Service); and Vaccine Victims Support Group. Some of the groups focus on one vaccine, especially MMR, and others are more radical in questioning the use of all vaccines. Given this, terms such as 'anti-vaccination movement' are misleading. The term 'Vaccine Critical groups' is therefore preferable. The research revealed that, as well as functioning as regular sources for journalists covering the vaccine issue, the groups also provide advice and support for their members, and for wider groups of parents who access their websites and other campaign materials.

The founders or coordinators of the Vaccine Critical groups were initially contacted by letter. These were then followed up with emails and phone calls where necessary. Two of the interviews were conducted over the telephone and the remainder at the home of the individual. The interview schedule was semi-structured but was carefully designed to allow the interviewee maximum space to pursue several issues. Given the aim of investigating how risk is constructed, questions were not asked directly about MMR or about risk/benefit calculations. Instead the groups were asked very broad questions such as 'What is your organization's policy towards childhood vaccination?' and 'What factors do you think influence a parent's decision about whether to have their child vaccinated?' I was thus very conscious of the dangers of closing off other analytical possibilities by assuming that risk is the dominant framework (Gofton and Haimes 1999).

The analysis of interview transcripts was carried out in conjunction with small-scale documentary analysis of written materials from the groups, including leaflets, magazines, and websites. All data were treated as discourse (Howarth 2000), notwithstanding the awareness that written text and interview data are produced differently. Indeed, it is recognized that there are multiple dimensions to the interview encounter. Insights from feminist and other literatures have helped make sense of some aspects of my personal research experience. One aspect of this experience is now briefly discussed.

During the interviews the leaders of the groups appeared not only to want to persuade me of their rationality and demonstrate their own 'moral adequacy' (Murphy and Dingwall 2003: 98), but also to believe that, through the interview, the terms of the debate could somehow be changed. If they could just convince me of the logic of their position, then my research would echo this and impact positively on the vaccination controversy. In reflecting on their own research, Bondi (2005) and Jarzabkowski (2001) also recount similar experiences.

To some extent, this experience is arguably an implicit part of most qualitative research. However, it is perhaps heightened for those studying an issue that has a high media or policy profile. Scott and colleagues describe this graphically in their phrase 'captive of controversy', used to describe what happens when the researcher is co-opted into the scientific (or risk) controversy they are trying to study (Scott *et al.* 1990). The implication of this argument is that those studying risk debates should be particularly aware of the need to manage interviewee expectations, where appropriate, and be clear about the objectives of their research. In some cases, influencing public debate in a certain direction may indeed be part of the research aims. In all cases, however, it should be remembered that those interviewed also inevitably have their own aims and perspectives. The broader point to make is that the social context in which research takes place – in my case periods of intense media interest in MMR – impacts on the lived experience of studying health, risk and vulnerability.

Risk discourses

The analysis involved investigating whether and how risk was discussed: this was defined broadly as including reference to probability, chance, harm or danger. The analysis reveals that risk is constructed in five different ways by the Vaccine Critical groups. These will now be discussed in turn and links made to existing literature, before wider conclusions are drawn.

Risk as unknowns

Not surprisingly, perhaps, vaccination promotion strategies do not generally utilize the idea of unknowns. In contrast, reference to uncertainty and unknowns is a central part of the Vaccine Critical discourse. There are different strands to this argument. First, there is criticism of the perceived short-termism of vaccine safety trials and the inadequate monitoring of vaccine reactions. This means that the 'true risk' of vaccination, in terms of their negative effects, remains unknown. This is exemplified in the following quote from the Informed Parent website: 'Q. Are there any reliable figures to compare complications of a disease with complications from a vaccine? No. Most vaccine reactions go unreported and are usually dismissed as a coincidence.'

Citing a *British Medical Journal* (BMJ) article as a way of implying legitimacy, JABS stresses that the size of vaccine safety trials, as well as their duration, is problematic:

And it's published in medical journals in the BMJ saying that pre-licensed trials are too small to show up the rare events, so you are relying on the monitoring system and when the monitoring system doesn't work because doctors say it's nothing to do with the vaccine, it doesn't get put forward for investigation.

(JABS)

In addition to this type of argument a wider discourse is also visible which relates to a more fundamental human ignorance about the body and the meaning and determinants of health and disease. The Informed Parent and vaccination.co.uk websites use very similar language posing straightforward and basic sounding questions, to which the answer is given that we simply don't know. The implication is that it is fruitless to try and rationally compare the benefits or risks of disease and vaccines:

1   How do vaccines affect the nervous system on a cellular level?
     No one knows.
2   How do vaccines cause damage on a cellular level?
     No one knows.

(vaccination.co.uk website)

During the interview, the Informed Parent expressed the idea that, fundamentally, we do not understand about the body: 'And I think the more you read on it, the more you realize what little we know about the body and health. There's so much we still don't understand.' This latter argument has implications beyond vaccination and is related to wider questions about faith in scientific knowledge and progress. Further discussion of this is unfortunately beyond the scope of this chapter. However, in terms of risk, the important point is that the groups describe a situation where the actual risk or impact of vaccination remains unknown. This discourse is evident in different forms but, taken as a whole, is starkly opposed to the certainty that risk statistics are supposed to imply (Petersen and Lupton 1996: 38). In other words, by concentrating on unknowns and uncertainties, the Vaccine Critical groups seek to undermine the value and relevance of official risk discourses.

Risk as individualized

Mass vaccination is justified through the theory of herd immunity, which promises benefits for the whole community. The Vaccine Critical groups express some concern with the utilitarian nature of mass vaccination. For example, JABS argues that proponents of the system know there will be individual casualties but believe that 'the system can mop them up', for the benefit of the community:

The majority – they probably will be fine, but it's the blow to the minority and when you are vaccinating half a million children a year the Department of Health can afford one or two casualties. But parents can't.

(JABS)

Very similar language, which expresses moral outrage at the way mass vaccination and policy makers conceptualize the individual, is used by VAN: 'The individual doesn't really matter. They know damn well that out of X million people they vaccinate a certain percentage do get side effects.' Despite these important exceptions, the Vaccine Critical groups do not primarily discursively present themselves as defenders of the individual. Rather, they aim to criticize vaccination, or conventional health care more generally, for treating everyone the same. For example, the web homepage of vaccination.co.uk makes this point: 'What may be right for one child could invariably be wrong for another.' A similar point is made in an article written for a VAN publication: 'We are all different from each other...Standard vaccinations take no account of the genetic diversity of individuals...Apart from true twins we are all different. That is the first cause of risk.'

The groups suggest different solutions to this problem. Some groups (AiA, JABS, Vaccine Victims) argue that a test should be developed to screen out genetically vulnerable babies who would not then be subject to the recommended vaccine schedule. This represents a technical solution to the problem of risk. For other groups, this would be wholly insufficient. For these latter groups, vaccination, far from symbolizing the community good, is itself an individualizing or privatizing strategy. This argument is made most clearly by vaccination.co.uk. They claim that, although, on the surface, the concept of herd immunity can be seen as supporting the community or even conforming to 'socialist' ideals, in practice vaccination is 'just an elastoplast over social problems'. Problems of ill health are conceptualized as social in nature and require significant state involvement. This is argued in light of a radio interview with a health professional who pointed to deaths from measles in Ireland as evidence for the need for continued vaccination:

So it's pretty much a social issue. So going back to the radio, the guy was talking about these kids in Ireland and everybody is getting scared, they are saying measles is a killer – see, proof. I would be arguing the proof is that governments don't want to invest in the inner cities and provide better housing. These families that might be on, whatever, unemployment, social security, they can't afford decent nutrition, not really educated so they prioritize the colour TV over vegetables. This is the society we have created...

(vaccination.co.uk)

What underlies this controversial argument is a particular view of health and disease. Whether an individual will get a disease is influenced by social factors (education, housing, diet), rather than vaccine status. The appropriate solution to the risk posed by disease is therefore social in nature, or more social than vaccine technology. The founder of the Informed Parent also argues that overall health status (including nutrition) will influence the likelihood of vaccine damage, although this, she stresses, is her personal opinion:

> Well, my personal opinion is that...we are all damaged. But many of us, because we've got reasonable health, we can tolerate a certain number of vaccines, so some of us might have quite a number. And I don't think that, you might not see any obvious signs of damage, but who's to say how healthy we would have been if we hadn't?
>
> (Informed Parent)

These data are complex to analyse but all relate to the social distribution of risk. The groups share the argument that the risk (of catching a disease, suffering complications from a disease, or even suffering an adverse reaction to a vaccine) is not distributed equally or randomly but is partly determined by individual genetic differences or social inequality. In practice, this argument challenges the value for the individual parent of risk statistics put out by the Department of Health. This relates to the wider problem about how to design health care messages for the whole population.

More fundamentally, the construction of risk as non-random and non-equal also represents a challenge to the *policy* of vaccinating all individuals. This does not support the argument, made by a regional director of public health, that vaccine critics are guilty of 'rampant individualism' (Ashton 2004), or ignoring the community benefits of herd immunity. Rather, it is the one-size-fits-all nature of mass vaccination that is being criticized. By recognizing that health and disease are influenced by several factors, the Vaccine Critical groups are in line with government health care messages in other areas, for example in coronary heart disease (CHD). Davison and colleagues (Davison *et al.* 1991) found that expert discourses relate CHD candidacy to factors such as diet, whereas lay epidemiology recognized the role of 'luck' in accounting for individual experience. In the vaccination domain, the data suggest the opposite: the dominant discourse claims that all children are at risk of disease, whereas the Vaccine Critical groups insist that risk factors are influential. Indeed, the image of the individual, each with their own mix of risk factors, is actually consistent with modern discourses of the 'new public health' that has emerged since the 1970s (Lupton 1995; Petersen and Lupton 1996). This point will be returned to later in the conclusion.

Risk as strategy: the role of fear

As discussed above, the Vaccine Critical groups tend to emphasize the unknowns that are associated with risk. Conversely, the groups also argue that risk is known but is concealed, manipulated or exaggerated by certain actors. This contrasts with the dominant vaccination discourse which assumes that risk statistics are neutral and objective. The critical discourse is used in two complementary ways: first through claiming that the actual risk of vaccine adverse events is being hidden from the public – the language here is about concealment versus transparency; second, by arguing that the risk associated with childhood diseases is being manipulated. For example, JABS explicitly claims that public risk perception is being deliberately heightened:

> We started off with drug manufacturers producing vaccines against the really serious illnesses like diphtheria, like tetanus, like polio, and then, because they can produce vaccines they are doing, and you've got to change the public's perception of that illness to change the product.
>
> (JABS)

What is fascinating about this data is the way that *fear* is constructed as a resource, used deliberately by government and the medical profession to change public perception. In the following extract, JFAVDC describes a kind of model, with distinct phases. In this model, a vaccine is developed against a disease and then risk statistics are produced to create public concern. This in turn results in public demand or acceptance of the new vaccine. In this example, JFAVDC refer to the possibility of introducing a chicken pox vaccine into the national recommended schedule (see BBC News 2002).

> I wonder why they are suddenly worrying about chickenpox, for instance. People have had chickenpox for hundreds of years...and there has never been any publicity from the Department [of Health] about 'this is a terrible disease and it kills hundreds of people every year'. But if they put out the vaccine for it within a month they have produced the figures 'thousands of children died last year' [laughs]...Whether they think people are stupid or what I don't know.
>
> (Justice for All Vaccine Damaged Children)

More broadly, fear is also discussed as part of the wider context of vaccination.

> I think fear has actually driven a lot of policies...Fear of the Public Health Laboratory and the government that they are not seen to be doing the best by the parents and children, fear of the parents not to do the best by their children, and fear of death.
>
> (AiA)

The Vaccine Critical groups who use this kind of discourse make clear that their aim is not to contribute to this climate of fear by scaring parents about the dangers associated with vaccines. Rather, the best case scenario is of a parent who feels confident enough to question the need for vaccination. For the Informed Parent, for example, fear is 'not a good place to be':

But there's always going to be a certain number that are scared of the vaccine side effects and they'll just not do it [vaccinate] because of that, and they'll just think 'oh, I'll take my chances' and that is not a good frame of mind to be in because you are always going to be panicking whatever...the fear thing is not a good place to be. You've got to really know why and what you're doing otherwise you will just get scared all the time and panic.

(Informed Parent)

This section has discussed the data which constructs risk as known but concealed and manipulated by those aiming to promote vaccination compliance. Here, risk and fear are conceptualized as strategies. This is in contrast to the assumptions in realist approaches, discussed earlier in the chapter, where risk, or more accurately risk statistics, are seen as objective representations of reality. This is not to say, of course, that the groups would necessarily identify themselves as taking a social constructionist line on risk. Indeed, by drawing a distinction between true risk and public risk perception they are implicitly supporting a realist approach. To clarify, the main point to be taken from this section is that risk is constructed as a political strategy, rather than objective or neutral, and this represents a significant challenge to the supposed authority of risk comparisons that are dominant in health and vaccination promotion campaigns (Hobson-West 2003).

Challenging the narrative of success

As highlighted at the start, vaccination is hailed as a highly successful technology by the public health and medical professions. This section reports on the data which show how the groups challenge the benefits or need for vaccination, rather than concentrating on the risks or dangers associated with it. There are two main ways in which this discourse is constructed: by challenging claims to historical success, and by questioning the underlying aim of disease eradication. It should be stressed that not all of the groups would use these discourses and challenge the view that vaccination has been responsible for a dramatic decline in infectious disease. However, four of the more 'radical' groups – vaccination.co.uk, VAN, Informed Parent and Vaccination Information – make this an important part of their argument.

First, some groups claim that other factors, such as diet, sanitation and mass education, explain historical increases in life expectancy. On this account, to credit vaccination is a 'blatant rewriting of history' (Vaccination Information, *open letter*). In the interview, Vaccination Information suggest why vaccination is so important to the medical profession as a symbol of success:

The medical professional cannot, does not shout about cancer and heart disease – look what a wonderful job we are doing. What they do say is if it wasn't for us you'd all be dying of...[infectious diseases]. Take away that as well and say 'that had zip to do with you'...they've got nothing...They are living on a reputation that isn't theirs.

(Vaccination Information)

Second, and even more controversially, some of the groups suggest that we should not necessarily aim to prevent childhood disease. Here the underlying rationale of vaccination is being challenged, and not efficacy. Discourses of alternative health are implicit in many of these arguments. For example, the Informed Parent states: 'You may decide that contracting measles will play a beneficial role, resulting in priming and maturing your child's immune system' (Informed Parent, website). In a similar vein, vaccination.co.uk imply that the contraction of natural measles may in fact be beneficial. Natural immunity, it is claimed, is 100% effective whereas vaccine induced immunity is not. The following quote implies frustration with the notion of risk as probability – 'the likelihood of measles' – and the preference for a more holistic view of health, where health is conceptualized as something broader than simply the absence of measles:

So if you want to vaccinate my children I want to know. I couldn't care less about the likelihood of measles, because I know my children have a strong immune system. I want to know can you tell me? Are they going to be healthier because they have been vaccinated? And to me that is the simple question. That is the only question the government should be asking.

(vaccination.co.uk)

In summary, the more radical of the Vaccine Critical groups challenge the narrative of success that is an important part of the pro-vaccination discourse. This is significant in that, by questioning the rationale for disease eradication and by challenging the received version of history, questions of relative risk are relegated to secondary importance. This evidence challenges the view that those who criticize vaccination have forgotten the benefits of vaccination and therefore overestimate risks (e.g. Bedford and Elliman 1998). Given that their aim is precisely to challenge the standard version of history, such statements are greeted with anger and frustration by some of the Vaccine Critical groups. Although risk and benefit are supposedly two sides of the same coin, I would argue that research with too narrow a focus on risk might miss these arguments. Admittedly, further studies would be needed to ascertain whether these discourses are used by a wider population of parents. However, research in another area is potentially relevant. The PABE report on attitudes to GM food in Europe concludes that resistance to the technology was partly about a failure to demonstrate *need* and not about cost/benefit calculations (Marris *et al.* 2001). Risk, in other words, is not the only measure by which technology is evaluated.

Further vaccine-related risks

Given the intensity of media debate at the time of the research, it did not come as a surprise that the issue of MMR and autism emerged as an important topic. When asked whether AAA has a policy towards vaccination, and whether this is a fair question, the leader responded:

> Unfortunately it is a fair question because that in a sense is what brought us together in the first place, a common belief that vaccination was deeply implicated in what had happened to these children. I don't think we could ever deny that.
>
> (AAA)

The reason that autism is not currently recognized as a vaccine risk is explained by this group as a result of ineffectual testing and monitoring. This goes back to the discussion of risk as unknowns at the start of the chapter. However, detailed analysis of the interview transcripts reveals that the subject of autism is placed in a wider pre-existing discourse, once again with links to alternative health, about the apparent rise of chronic conditions in the West. The groups explain this rise as a response to the suppression of the immune system, partially caused by vaccination. JABS puts it very succinctly:

> Fair enough we want to try and eradicate these diseases but at what cost?...We can't exchange acute conditions for chronic conditions. Just try and stop the child catching measles but give them epilepsy instead, but at what cost?
>
> (JABS)

Another of the groups makes a similar point:

> There is no doubt that a child with a weakened immune system is at greater risk from infectious diseases, than a healthy child, but there is no evidence that vaccinations make people healthier. On the contrary it is most likely that we have traded what were normal childhood illnesses 40 years ago, for normal childhood diseases today such as asthma, eczema, and allergies.
>
> (vaccination.co.uk)

The more 'radical' of the Vaccine Critical groups even link vaccination to wider social problems. For example, VAN discusses the claim that vaccination has been linked with fertility problems in the developing world. The Informed Parent implicates vaccines in causing behavioural problems beyond the field of health:

> Even neurologically if it's affecting people, subtle damage, people can't even think straight. I'm not one for saying that everything out there that's a

problem is to do with vaccination. But vaccination could be, could be linked to all these different aspects.

(Informed Parent)

The data are unclear as to whether these groups actively promote such 'conspiracy theories' or whether they merely wish to report them as part of a wider critical discourse that is available on other websites. In both examples cited, the leaders refer to published books where such arguments are said to originate, perhaps as a way of distancing themselves from ideas they recognize to be highly controversial. The 'could be, could be' in the last quote is also a way of stressing uncertainty.

Overall, this final section has discussed how the groups refer to 'further risks' or negative consequences of vaccination. For anxious public health officials this could be taken as concrete evidence that Vaccine Critical groups advertise 'unproven' risks of vaccination. However, as has been shown in this chapter, this is only *one part* of the discourse of Vaccine Critical groups who also focus on unknowns, the distribution of risk, risk as strategy and the reliability of historical success narratives. Furthermore, the risks that are discussed in this final section, of autism and other chronic conditions, are not even officially recognized as vaccine risks. From the point of view of the Vaccine Critical groups, therefore, tables of risk comparisons used by the government remain irrelevant in their capacity to accurately represent the choice that parents face.

Conclusions

The aim of this chapter was to investigate the discourses of Vaccine Critical groups in the UK. A constructionist approach was adopted in order to analyse how ideas about risk are formulated and framed. The underlying theoretical assumption is that deeming something a risk (and then managing or communicating about it) is not merely a technical matter but is a result of a social and political process. The implication is that opposition to expert risk discourses is not about a technical misunderstanding. Resistance can instead be studied as a critical response to the way in which risk is formulated and constructed by the dominant expert discourse.

As predicted by existing literature on other topics (Wynne 1992; Marris *et al.* 2001), unknowns emerged as an important discourse. Sometimes these unknowns are temporary and could in principle be resolved by further research (or different monitoring or regulatory systems). At other times, however, there is reference to a more profound collective ignorance about the causes of health and disease. In this latter case, uncertainty is not something to be transcended or translated into certainty (Zinn 2006). Either way, existing risk information is seen as insufficient. Risk is also constructed as non-objective and strategic: politics and science are therefore closely entangled. By questioning the one-size-fits-all nature of mass vaccination, current policy is being criticized but so is the ability of epidemiology to recognize and account for individual differences. Questioning the contribution of vaccination in reducing death and disease amounts to challenging the standard version of history and the success claims for vaccine technology. Taken together, what these discourses demonstrate is a fundamental reframing of risk but also a problematization of faith in science and professional expertise. The data thus confirms the close relationship between risk and trust (Wynne 1993; Alaszewski 2003; Hobson-West 2007).

On a more theoretical level, some wider conclusions can be drawn. On the one hand, the MMR controversy could be analysed as empirical evidence for, or cultural expression of, life in a risk society. For Beck and those who have adopted his thesis, risk is a key principle of modern society, rather than simply one element of it, and 'debates and conflicts over risks have begun to dominate public, political and private realms' (Lupton 1999: 59). Debate over MMR and childhood vaccination would be easily identified as one of these risk conflicts. In risk society, what may at first appear to be a technical matter can become the subject of fierce public debate (Moore 2003). In addition, autism and vaccine reactions could be categorized as Beck's human-made risks, in contrast to the natural disasters more associated with a previous epoch. Furthermore, if there is a widespread parental fear around vaccination issues, then this could be interpreted as evidence for a heightened level of social anxiety (Wilkinson 2001; Brownlie and Howson 2006). In short, therefore, the value of the risk society approach appears to be confirmed through an analysis of the MMR issue.

On the other hand, Beck famously argued that 'smog is democratic' (Beck 1992: 36) to highlight how contemporary risks (such as the risk associated with nuclear power) have the potential to affect everyone, regardless of social status, place or nationality. However, as has been demonstrated, the Vaccine Critical groups make their case by maintaining that risks to health (from diseases or from vaccines) are explicitly *not* distributed equally or randomly but are influenced by several factors. These factors vary and include genetics and lifestyle, that are important for the 'new public health', and older issues of structural inequality. In this respect at least, the relevance of the risk society thesis, for capturing the vaccination debate, is challenged. This is a topic that undoubtedly deserves further empirical and theoretical analysis. Overall, the contribution of this chapter is to highlight the importance of risk, both for justifying vaccination policy and for vaccination resistance. The discussion also shows that teasing out understandings of risk is not merely an academic preoccupation. In practice, reframing risk is a political strategy that enables opponents to undermine powerful discourses that support hegemonic policies, such as mass childhood vaccination.

References

Alaszewski, A. (2003) 'Risk, trust and health', *Health, Risk and Society* 5(3): 235–9.

Annandale, E. (1998) *The Sociology of Health and Medicine: A Critical Introduction.* Cambridge: Polity Press.

Ashton, J. (2004) Interview, in *You and Yours.* BBC Radio 4. January 21.

Bauer, M. (1995) 'Towards a functional analysis of resistance', in M. Bauer (ed.) *Resistance to New Technology.* Cambridge: Cambridge University Press.

BBC News (2002) *MMR Superjab Planned*. 15 February. Online. Available at http://news.bbc.co.uk/1/hi/health/1823248.stm (accessed 6 March 2006).

BBC News (2004) *Profile: Dr Andrew Wakefield*. 23 February. Online. Available at http://news.bbc.co.uk/1/hi/health/3513365.stm (accessed 1 August 2005).

Beck, U. (1992) *Risk Society: Towards a New Modernity*. London: Sage.

Bedford, H. and Elliman, D. (1998) *Childhood Immunisation: A Review*, vol. 1. London: Health Education Authority.

Bennett, P. (1999) 'Understanding responses to risk: Some basic findings', in P. Bennett and K. Calman (eds) *Risk Communication and Public Health*. Oxford: Oxford University Press.

Bondi, L. (2005) 'The place of emotions in research: From partitioning emotion and reason to the emotional dynamics of research relationships', in J. Davidson, L. Bondi and M. Smith (eds) *Emotional Geographies*. Aldershot: Ashgate.

Brown, T. (2000) 'AIDS, risk and social governance', *Social Science and Medicine* 50: 1273–84.

Brownlie, J. and Howson, A. (2005) 'Leaps of faith and MMR: An empirical study of trust', *Sociology* 39(4): 221–39.

Brownlie, J. and Howson, A. (2006) '"Between the demands of truth and government": Health practitioners, trust and immunisation work', *Social Science and Medicine* 62: 433–43.

Davison, C., Smith, G.D. and Frankel, S. (1991) 'Lay epidemiology and the prevention paradox: The implications of coronary candidacy for health education', *Sociology of Health and Illness* 13(1): 1–19.

Deer, B. (2004) 'Revealed: MMR research scandal', *The Sunday Times*, 22 February. Online. Available at http://briandeer.com/mmr/lancet-deer-1.htm (accessed 7 July 2005).

Department of Health (2004) *Full Immunisation Schedule*. Online. Available at http://www.immunisation.nhs.uk/article.php?id=97 (accessed 8 May 2006).

Dew, K. (1999) 'Epidemics, panic and power: Representations of measles and measles vaccines', *Health* 3: 379–98.

Ehreth, J. (2003) 'The global value of vaccination', *Vaccine* 21: 596–600.

Gofton, L. and Haimes, E. (1999) 'Necessary evils? Opening up closings in sociology and biotechnology', *Sociological Research Online* 4. Online. Available at http://www.socresonline.org.uk/4/3/gofton.html (accessed 19 September 2005).

Hargreaves, I., Lewis, J. and Speers, T. (2003) *Towards a Better Map: Science, the Public and the Media*. Swindon: ESRC.

Harrabin, R., Coote, A. and Allen, J. (2003) *Health in the News: Risk, Reporting and Media Influences*. London: Kings Fund Publishers.

Hobson-West, P. (2003) 'Understanding vaccination resistance: Moving beyond risk', *Health, Risk and Society* 5(3): 273–83.

Hobson-West, P. (2005) 'Understanding resistance to childhood vaccination in the UK: Radicals, reformists and the discourses of risk, trust and science', unpublished PhD thesis, University of Nottingham.

Hobson-West, P. (2007) '"Trusting blindly can be the biggest risk of all": Organised resistance to childhood vaccination in the UK', *Sociology of Health and Illness* 29: 198–215.

Hodge, J.G. and Gostin, L.O. (2003) 'School vaccination requirements: Historical, social and legal perspectives', *Kentucky Law Journal* 90: 831–90.

Howarth, D. (2000) *Discourse*. Buckingham: Open University Press.

Jarzabkowski, L. (2001) 'Emotional labour in educational research', *Queensland Journal of Educational Research* 17: 123–37. Online. Available at http://education.curtin.edu.au/iier/qjer/qjer17/jarzabkowski.html (accessed 19 September 2005).

Lupton, D. (1995) *The Imperative of Health: Public Health and the Regulated Body.* London: Sage.

Lupton, D. (1999) *Risk.* London: Routledge.

Marris, C., Wynne, B., Simmons, P. and Weldon, S. (2001) *Public Perceptions of Agricultural Biotechnology in Europe.* Final report of the PABE research project. Online. Available at http://csec.lancs.ac.uk/pabe/ (accessed 24 August 2007).

McGuire, C. (1998) *Health Update: Immunisation.* London: Health Education Authority.

Moore, A. (2003) 'Democracy and risk: The case of MMR', paper presented at the *Political Studies Association Conference*, University of Leicester, 15–17 April.

Murphy, E. and Dingwall, R. (2003) *Qualitative Methods and Health Policy Research.* New York: Aldine de Gruyter.

NHS (2004) *Welcome to MMR: The Facts.* Online. Available at http://www.mmrthefacts.nhs.uk/ (accessed 19 September 2005).

Petersen, A. and Lupton, D. (1996) *The New Public Health.* London: Sage.

Pidgeon, N., Kasperson, R.E. and Slovic, P. (2003) *The Social Amplification of Risk.* Cambridge: Cambridge University Press.

Poland, G.A. and Jacobson, R.M. (2001) 'Understanding those who do not understand: A brief review of the anti-vaccine movement', *Vaccine* 19: 2440–5.

Poltorak, M., Leach, M., Fairhead, J. and Cassell, J. (2005) 'MMR talk and vaccination choices: An ethnographic study in Brighton', *Social Science and Medicine* 61(3): 709–19.

Rayner, G. (2002) 'Panic sets in as disease dies out', The *Guardian*, 18 March.

Scott, P., Richards, E. and Martin, B. (1990) 'Captives of controversy: The myth of the neutral social researcher in contemporary scientific controversies', *Science, Technology and Human Values* 15: 474–94.

Spier, R.E. (2001) 'Perceptions of risk of vaccine adverse events: A historical perspective', *Vaccine* 20: S78–S84.

Streefland, P. (2001) 'Public doubts about vaccination safety and resistance against vaccination', *Health Policy* 55: 159–72.

Wakefield, A.J., Murch, S.H., Anthony, S., Linnell, J., Casson, D.M., Malik, M. *et al.* (1998) 'Ileal-lymphoid-nodular hyperplasia, non-specific colitis, and pervasive developmental disorder in children', *Lancet* 352: 637–41.

Wilkinson, I. (2001) *Anxiety in a Risk Society.* London: Routledge.

Wynne, B. (1992) 'Uncertainty and environmental learning: Reconceiving science and policy in the preventive paradigm', *Global Environmental Change* 2: 111–27.

Wynne, B. (1993) 'Public uptake of science: A case for institutional reflexivity', *Public Understanding of Science* 2: 321–37.

Zinn, J. (2006) 'Recent developments in sociology of risk and uncertainty', *Forum: Qualitative Sozialforschung/ Qualitative Social Research* 7(1), art. 30. Online. Available at http://www.qualitative-research.net/fqs-texte/1-06/06-1-30-e.htm (accessed 10 May 2006).

Index